The Vibrant Life

The Vibrant Life

Simple Meditations to Use Your Energy Effectively

Donna Thomson

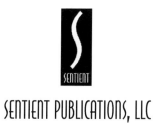

SENTIENT PUBLICATIONS, LLC

First Sentient Publications edition 2006
Cover design by Kim Johansen
Cover art by Robert Sturman Studio
Book design by Rudy Ramos

A paperback original

This information contained in this book is intended only as a guide and not as a substitute for professional medical help.

Library of Congress Cataloging-in-Publication Data

Thomson, Donna.
  The vibrant life : simple meditations to use your energy effectively / Donna Thomson.
    p. cm.
  ISBN 1-59181-046-9
  1. Meditation. 2. Vitality. I. Title.
  BF637.M4T46 2006
      158.1'28—dc22
                              2005033900

Printed in the United States of America

10 9 8 7 6 5 4 3

SENTIENT PUBLICATIONS, LLC
1113 Spruce Street
Boulder, CO 80302
www.sentientpublications.com

This book is dedicated to the deepest intention and
highest potential of each reader.

Do you know
you are all stars and flowers,
a gathering of petals,
a radiant dispersal of light?

Do you know
you are a golden thread woven into intricate image,
a tapestry forever spinning itself anew?

Do you know
you are pure love
for everything that is—
for what you are?

DONNA THOMSON

Table of Contents

Introduction

THIS BOOK IS BASED ON A FEW SIMPLE PREMISES:

- One of the most important things you can do for your physical, emotional, and spiritual health is to pay attention to your energy, learn to understand it, work with it, conserve it, and use it effectively.

- Your state of mind affects your energy level. It is possible to increase your personal energy by using your mind. The meditations, visualizations, and active imagination exercises in this book are designed to help you do exactly that.

- You don't have a lot of time. You may not want another program or regimen that promises success if you can do it every day for a week, a month, or forever. The mental exercises in this book can be done at your own pace. They are intended for use as you feel the need for them. Many of them take only a few minutes and can be done almost anywhere, anytime.

- Everybody has energy, because everybody *is* energy. Many biologists and physicists have conducted experiments demonstrating that human beings and their environment constitute one vibrant, coherent energy field.[1] The very first chapter of this book is designed to help you experience that you are energy. People often say, "I don't have enough energy." Once you experience that you and the world around you are energy, that energy is the very nature and essence of your being, you can no longer say that. When you let go of the idea of having or not having, you open the door into a field of abundant energy. If you have experienced a chronic state of low energy for a long time, and feel you don't even have the energy to do the exercises in this book, read the chapter "Breaking the Downward Cycle" first.

• There is no such thing as a formula that works all the time for everybody. Each person is unique, and what helps one may not help another. What helps you one day may not help you at another time. What helped somebody two thousand years ago might not work in the modern world. The meditations, visualizations, and active imagination exercises in this book are synthesized from many spiritual, metaphysical, and psychotherapeutic traditions, as well as from my own healing work with people. You can choose what works for you from day to day. Read the whole book from start to finish, and then decide which exercises you want to begin with. Or read first whatever chapters attract you most.

If you work through the book from the beginning, you will find that the exercises are designed to steadily build your skills in working with your energy. The exercises begin with helping you to conserve your energy, calm it, nurture it with the breath, cleanse it, recharge it, and protect it. You will then go on to working with other people's energies in difficult situations. Exercises that help you develop greater awareness, experience the power of choice, and shift your thought patterns provide the foundation for clearing old patterns that obstruct the free flow of your energy. Then there are several meditations to help you connect with the positive, nourishing energies in yourself, the world, and the universe.

As you read, play with the exercises. Explore them. Use them as you need to. As soon as something becomes a formula, a way, or a method, it becomes fixed. As soon as it becomes fixed, it loses energy. Energy is change, movement, fluidity, and flexibility. Use these meditations however you choose, but please don't turn them into a fixed program—a "should."

- The imagination is a powerful tool for change. We have lost an enormous amount of energy in today's world by closing the door on the imagination, by channeling it only into what is defined as productive activity, in discounting vision and dream as daydreaming. These meditations are intended to reawaken the imagination, to arouse the energy lying dormant in the suppressed imagination. Very often, traditional methods of meditation—not to mention traditional methods of parenting and education—direct people to repress their imaginations. People are warned not to let their minds wander, to pay attention, whether it is to a math problem or to a spiritual practice. The mind wants to wander. If it is allowed to wander, with a little guidance and a few maps, it releases huge amounts of energy. It brings visions and the energy to act on the visions. So in this book we will wander together in a world not so visible, not so known. The book is a map to the edge of the map, after which you're on your own, creating your own incomparable journey.

- The meditations offered in this book are not intended to take you out of yourself into some other reality. They are meant to take you deeper into yourself and your life and to help you live in this amazingly complex, wonderful, and yet sometimes terrifying world. They are tools intended to help you build that most mysterious of structures: a conscious self. This is a self that is more than the product of old conditioning, more than the self that is created by parents, ancestors, and society. It is a self we create. We cannot deny or eliminate the past, our history. But we can work with it, make conscious choices in relation to it, and thereby give birth to ourselves. Again, to bring life into being requires energy. These meditations are intended to give you greater access to the life force so you may continue to create yourself.

This book is not about defining energy or understanding it from a conceptual or scientific point of view. There are countless books you can read about the nature of energy. You can learn about energy from spiritual teachers and modern physicists.

Fundamentally, energy is one of the simplest things in the world to experience. You know when you have it and when you don't. You know when it's flowing and when it isn't. That's the kind of energy this book is about: the energy most people feel they don't have enough of these days; the life energy you feel flowing in you when you begin to recover from an illness, after an exercise session, when you're in love, whenever you're fully involved in what you're doing. This book is about how to have more of the energy it takes to accomplish what you want to do, to live the life you want to live. It has a purely practical orientation. The Buddha once said that if you encounter a man with an arrow in him, you don't spend a lot of time discussing how the arrow got there or what kind of arrow it is. You pull out the arrow and tend the wound. So whatever blocks you experience to the free flow and expression of your energy, this book is about helping you remove them.

As the modern world grows ever more stressful, we have to understand that meditations such as the ones in this book are not a luxury. We need inner strength, peace, awareness, and lots of energy to find our way in today's world. This book provides exercises to help you find your inner compass and trust it.

Both modern science and ancient wisdom teach us that everything is interconnected in the great web of life.[2] Chief Seattle's often-quoted statement that what we do to the web, we do to ourselves,[3] is also true in reverse: what we do to ourselves, we do to the web. This means that as we tend to ourselves with care, attention, and understanding, the effect ripples outward. As we learn to work with our energy—to understand it, conserve it, and use it effectively—we not only develop our inner resources, we also become more aware of how we use the resources in our environment. We experience greater peace in ourselves and in our immediate surroundings. As we experience greater balance in our own lives, we bring greater balance to the world in which we live.

So this book is about pulling arrows and reweaving the web, about finding your compass and living consciously in a stressful world. It's about experiencing the abundant energy that is your essential nature. May that experience bring health, harmony, and balance into your life and the lives of those around you.

A Few Words
About Meditation

THE MENTAL EXERCISES IN THIS BOOK UTILIZE A VARIETY OF MEDITATION, visualization, and active imagination techniques. Many people experience a block about meditation; they think they can't do it. If you are one of these people, please don't be intimidated by this word. I find there are four common misconceptions about meditation that make it more difficult for people.

Misconception number one: You have to be disciplined to meditate. Meditation should be done for a certain amount of time every day. You should sit in a certain way. You should have one practice and stick to it.

For some people, this approach to meditation works. If it does, that's great. If it doesn't, don't decide that meditation is not for you. People lead hectic lives and the pace is increasing. For people with families, full-time jobs, demanding schedules, it can be almost impossible to fit in even a half hour a day of meditation. And these people can certainly use the extra energy given by meditation!

Meditation can be woven into your day, in moments here and there: at your desk, in between errands, in the line at the bank. Close your eyes, focus on your breath, and practice any one of the methods you will find in this book. Open your eyes, and it's like you've had a bath, a cool drink on a hot day, a little journey to another state of being. Meditative time is not the same as "real time." A few seconds of meditation can give you as much energy as a night's sleep or a cup of coffee. It can be helpful to have periods of retreat—an afternoon, a day, or a week that you set aside for being quiet and reflective—but it isn't essential. We live in a sound-byte world, where our days are often fragmented and chaotic. Attention spans are short. Instead of fighting this, we can gain more energy and become less tense by accepting it. You can move in and out of a meditative state in a matter of seconds.

This brings us to *misconception number two:* The state of calm and peace you may experience at times when you meditate is something you should always feel when you meditate, and, not only that, you should feel it all the rest of the time too. If you meditate, you will never yell at your kids or spouse. You will never get angry at your boss. If you do, there's something wrong with your meditation, or meditation isn't working for you and isn't worth doing.

This is like thinking that because you're going to get hungry again, there's no point in eating. Day and night, we experience constant, shifting states of consciousness. If we try to hang onto the nice ones and deny the painful or less comfortable ones, we end up tense, worried, self-judging, and generally unhappy. As you meditate, you will become familiar with a more grounded, centered, spacious state of consciousness. You won't be able to maintain it always. The habits of the mind are powerful, and so are external pulls and demands. To begin to experience a state of loving awareness and increased energy, to remember it, and to know the possibility of returning to it is the beauty of meditation.

Misconception number three is related to Number Two: The purpose of meditation is to calm the mind. Therefore, if you have a lot of thoughts, that's not good. Good meditation means having an empty mind with few thoughts.

There's no such thing as bad meditation. You can't fail at doing meditation. Of course, it's nice to experience a serene mind, empty of worries. It's wonderful to experience bliss and peace—a state of consciousness beyond the stresses and demands of daily life. These states are emphasized in many spiritual traditions in which people meditate to attain enlightenment. If you meditate for any length of time, especially in the framework of a spiritual tradition, you will experience these states. However, in their desire to attain a certain state of mind, a lot of people end up approaching meditation as a battle—a struggle with their own mind, their lack of discipline, their ego. It becomes another exercise in will.

It doesn't take much self-discipline and willpower to close your eyes for a couple of minutes periodically throughout the day. It takes *remembering*. It is about exercising your power of choice. I can either feel stressed, anxious, worried, and fatigued, or I can take a few minutes to enter another state of consciousness. It's up to me. Which do I choose? I choose for a few minutes to become centered, relaxed, and calm. I may soon find myself again worried and fatigued. That's okay. I gave myself a break. I experienced a different state. I exercised choice. It's important to highlight the change, the moment of calm that comes, rather than to despair over the return to the usual state of mind.

In any meditation, you will experience lots of thoughts, feelings, and distractions from the central practice. So be it. If meditation can give you the experience of not fighting yourself, of accepting what is at any given moment, then you already have more energy.

We waste a lot of energy in battling ourselves. You know yourself. You can find the meditations that are right for you. Some people need to focus and concentrate their minds; some people need to let their minds journey. Some days, you may need a meditation that helps you to focus; other days, you may need to wander. Trust yourself. The purpose of this book is to give you many options, lots of choices. Become familiar with the meditations, and you won't really even have to think about it. The right one for the right time will arise as necessary.

Many of the exercises in this book involve visualization. People often dismiss visualization, saying they can't see things in their mind; therefore, they can't do it. That's *misconception number four.*

Visualization doesn't mean you have to have a completely clear image in your mind. You can have a general sense, or impression, of what you are trying to see. Or you can simply tell yourself what is happening—*I am surrounding myself with light*—

and feel that it is happening. To visualize means to sense inwardly, to make real in your consciousness, what you want to experience in your day-to-day life. You can do this with images, words, or feelings.

Meditation is something you really can do to support your life and growth, to bring you joy, and to increase your energy. It can open the door to a new experience of yourself, a new way of seeing this universe, a new connection with all that is, and to a source of energy that is constantly flowing. Here is a simple meditation technique that forms the basis for many of the methods described in the following chapters. It is called simply, "Following the Breath."

Following the Breath

Sit down quietly and comfortably, or lie down if you choose. Close your eyes and become aware of your breath. Don't try to regulate it. Just become aware of it. Follow it with your mind as it moves in and out of the body. Notice the inhalation and the exhalation. Focus your attention on your breath, let your thoughts, feelings, the tensions of the day all be carried by the breath and dissolved away in it.

As the mind wanders—gets involved in thoughts about what you could be doing or should be doing—just gently return your attention to the breath when you remember to do so. That's it.

Do this for one minute, half an hour, or all day. Don't strain; don't tense up around the breath. Just relax. Enjoy the gift of your own breath bringing you energy.

You can experience this book as a guided meditation. The meditations are woven into the text as awareness weaves throughout our daily life. There is no separation. As you read the book, you are already meditating. Let yourself experience that. It's so simple. Just keep reading.

Working with Light

....

MANY OF THE MEDITATIONS WE WILL DO TOGETHER INVOLVE WORKING WITH light. Light is energy. Think about different qualities of light that you experience. There's a certain light that comes in the late afternoon in autumn, a mellow golden light full of peacefulness. There's dawn light, the lavender rose of the sky at sunrise. Midday brings bright and radiant light. Sometimes, light comes through a window in just such a way that when you see it, you feel a moment of wonder, a connection with something greater than yourself. The stars in the huge night sky awaken that wonder, that sense of presence. A rainbow shines with hope and promise. Sunlight filters through green leaves; when you lie beneath a tree in springtime, you feel touched by this light and healed.

In the meditations that follow, light represents healing energy—the creative life force. In the Bible, God looks out over the dark void and says, "Let there be light!" From that light, all creation comes into being. Light is a visible, tangible form of the energy that surrounds us, that we are made of. As we work with light, visualize it, imagine it, we connect consciously with that creative force.

Our human lives are a dance of light and dark, sunshine and shadow, creation and destruction. I do not present light here as a weapon to be used against darkness. The light I am speaking of illuminates and embraces the good and the bad, the weak and the strong, positive and negative states of being. It does not deny anger, sorrow, fear, or pain. What is called the dark has its own power. The night sky, the cave of the hermit, the womb of the mother: the dark is a place we go to dream, rest, and receive visions of light. In the Eastern traditions, this dance is called the yin and the yang—the receptive and the creative.

You can imagine that white light, often used by healers, is the pure light of creation. It is powerful, healing, and intense. It represents the universal energy. Then there are the colors of light, the rainbow spectrum that is the universal white light filtered through the prism of this world of form. Imagine that these colors of light feed you and nourish your energy just as food nourishes your physical body. Red and orange, yellow and green, blue and purple—each color of light has its own qualities, its own vibration. Experiment with them. We will use the full range of the spectrum in the meditations to come. I frequently also will use golden light. In my experience, golden light brings growth, transformation, and strength. It is the light of the sun, warmth, and life. It absorbs negative thoughts, washes away old fears, and tenderly embraces my most rigid belief systems. It helps put me in touch with my deepest self. For protection, balancing, and cleansing, I use rainbow light.

Please note that I am not asking you to believe anything—to accept anything as fact. I am especially not trying to engage in a scientific discussion of light and its energetic or healing properties. I am asking you to imagine. As you imagine yourself surrounded by light, nourished by light, and protected by light, you can experience a shift in your energy. Your understanding of what it means to work with light will be experiential, not theoretical.

You Are Energy

BEGIN BY REFLECTING ON THE WORD ENERGY. BREATHE IT IN AND FEEL THE word in you. What is energy? How do you experience it? Does the very word bring a flow of energy to you, or does it produce a feeling of fatigue and hopelessness? Just notice your responses. If you are used to feeling a lack of energy, you may feel frustrated as soon as you think about it. If this is so, it's important to shift your association with the word, the idea, of energy. Let yourself breathe in the possibility that you can experience more energy.

Prana

Sit down quietly, take a breath, be aware of that breath, and meditate for a few moments, following your breath. Imagine that with each breath, energy is coming into you, flowing through your body.

Prana is the Sanskrit word for life force, the energy that creates and sustains the entire universe. Experiment with using this word. As you breathe in, imagine yourself soaked in prana and permeated by prana. Feel the prana going to every corner of your body.

Use your imagination. As you breathe in the prana, the life force energy, imagine all that is going on in your body at this very moment. Your heart is beating; blood is flowing and pulsing. Nerve cells are transmitting impulses. Cells are dividing and dying. Food is being digested. Glands are secreting. Countless processes are occurring simultaneously within you as you sit here quietly breathing, reading these words.

Think of how much energy is working in you at this moment. Appreciate the energy of the blood, the cells, the heart, the liver, and the brain. Even if every part of the body isn't working optimally, you are still a vast storehouse of energy. Don't concentrate on what isn't there. Feel how much energy you must have simply to be here—alive, breathing, and reading this book.

Allow the thought *I am a vast storehouse of energy* to linger and reverberate in your mind. Know that as you explore the exercises in this book, you will discover how to access and replenish that storehouse.

Resolve to eliminate these phrases from your vocabulary:

"I don't have the energy."

"I don't have any energy."

"I don't have enough energy."

Instead, you can say, "I need to replenish my energy today." "I need to be careful with my energy today." "I need to help my energy flow more freely today." Remember that you always have energy, more than you think. Contemplate the fact, daily, that you are full of energy, in all the ways you have just experienced. Simply because you are alive, you are full of energy.

So, once again, breathe quietly, and go through your body, imagining the energy that is at work in every part of you. Finish with the affirmation *I am a vast storehouse of energy*. The human body is energy; it is inwardly in constant motion. The exercises in this book will help you to release the energy that is already there within you.

Setting Boundaries and Conserving Your Energy

IN OUR CULTURE TODAY, WE DON'T UNDERSTAND WHAT IT MEANS TO CONSERVE energy. Our society is built on expending—on energy going out and out. At a global level, we continue to drain the earth's resources. The United States has a trade deficit of billions of dollars. The health of our economy is defined by how much people spend. We are taught that if we want to succeed, we have to put out energy, work long hours, sacrifice our personal lives, and give it all we've got. People struggle with chronic fatigue, exhaustion, stress, and burnout. There are few models in our culture for conservation, restoration, and replenishment of resources. We are experiencing in our own lives the truth that what we do to the web, we do to ourselves. We have drained and exhausted the earth's resources and energy, and now we find ourselves drained and exhausted as well.

We don't seem to understand energy. We don't understand that the flow of energy operates on the principle of exchange: what you take out, you have to restore. I live in a house that operates entirely off the grid. All our electricity comes from the sun. We have a fairly modest system, and so I learned the principle of energy exchange very quickly. If I use a lot of power one cloudy day, I may have to wait for a few sunny days before I can watch a movie on my television, use my washing machine, or surf the net.

It's so simple. The same principle applies to me. I use my energy every day. I need to conserve my energy, take care of it, restore and replenish it, before I use more. Eating and sleeping alone will not accomplish this, especially since these days so many people eat on the run and sleep restlessly.

Take a moment and think about how much energy you use and expend in the course of a day. Think about the water you use, the electricity. Reflect on how much energy it takes to support your lifestyle, no matter how simple you may think it is. Do you have any idea how many watts of electricity your television uses every time you turn it on? Or the hair dryer, the toaster, or the stove? You may be appalled at the state of the world, but do you have any specific, tangible idea of how much you contribute each day to the ongoing, constant drain on our resources?

Reflect on your personal energy. Think about the energy that's used up in working, relating to people, doing errands, even having a good time. You may know you feel drained when you come home from work, but what is draining you? Do you have any idea how much of your personal energy you can lose through a chance encounter with another person—a coworker, parent, boss, spouse, or that neighbor who drives you crazy?

In a solar electrical system, there are meters that show you exactly how much power you are using when you turn on a computer, a light, or a power tool. Spend a day imagining that you are carrying around such a meter. What makes the numbers go up? What experiences give you energy? Where is your sunshine? What makes your energy plummet to dangerously low levels? If it's a "cloudy" day—one when you're feeling low anyway—a little drain can take you very low. How do you make some space in the sun for yourself? That is, how do you restore your energy?

If you take stock of your overall use of energy, you may find some small ways that you can conserve energy in the outer world. Get rid of a few appliances, carpool when you can, flush the toilet a little less often, buy fewer things, or plant a tree. There are countless small ways of disengaging from the larger system of energy outflow and unconscious energy loss. These are important, but it can sometimes be difficult to experience the effect of such action on the global situation. However, if you also begin to pay attention to your use of your inner energy, you will find that your personal day-to-day experience of life can change. You may actually experience more energy.

A great deal of energy gets drained in our interactions with other people. Certainly, we have relationships that energize us, in which we experience a wonderful exchange of energy. However, almost everyone I encounter also has relationships they experience as draining; it's just a fact of human existence that for certain encounters, we need to know how to conserve and replenish our energy.

People talk a lot about setting boundaries these days; this is a necessary skill if one is to conserve one's energy and not allow it to be drained by other people. However, few of us have been taught to do this. The following exercise is simple and effective, and it will teach you how to tangibly create a boundary for yourself in relationship to others. It turns your attention to your energy. It preserves and conserves your energy, keeping it available to support your life. It does not isolate you and cut you off from human interaction; rather it provides a different basis for relationship, one in which you are thoroughly grounded in yourself. Regularly practiced, this exercise prevents other people from pulling on and draining your energy. Once you have practiced it for a while, you can do it in three seconds if necessary.

The Golden Line

Sit down quietly the first few times you do this exercise. Later, you can do it anywhere—while you are engaged in conversation, standing on the bus or train, sitting at your desk. For now, sit down and breathe quietly, calming the energy for a few moments. Read the meditation through first, and then try it.

Imagine that you are drawing a line of golden light around your body with your mind. Begin at the top of the head, a few inches out from your body. Bring the line down the right side of the head, down the neck and shoulder and arm, around every finger, back up the right arm, down the right side of the body, along the outside of the right leg, around every single toe, back up the inside of the right leg, and so on, around the body and back up to the top of the head.

This is a single unbroken line. If you lose it, start over. If you notice tension or obstruction, just continue on. This is not a hazy cloud of light surrounding you. This is a precise, defined line. It outlines the body like a two-dimensional drawing on a blackboard.

My experience with this exercise is that it's most helpful to draw the line fairly close—two to four inches out from the body. If you have a different experience, do what feels right to you. Remember, though, that this exercise is not about surrounding yourself with light for protection. (For that, see the chapter on "Psychic Protection.") This is about self-definition, drawing the outline of your unique self as a cartographer would delineate the borders of a country on a map. If you try to define too large an area, you can lose that sense of boundary.

Once you have drawn the line all the way around, sit quietly and feel it; imagine it as the border, the boundary, of your unique and personal being. Any influence from the outside may enter only if invited. Imagine that you feel your own personal energy flowing from the top of your head down through your body, into your legs, and back up again. It is like the blood circulating in your body. You are experiencing the flow of your own life energy in your energy system—your field. Feel the energy flowing within the vessel you have defined. Do this for as long as you like.

Finally, return to the line of light and redraw it, with the intention that it accompany you as you go out into the world. Thank the life energy for its support; honor it as it flows within you. It's a good idea to follow this meditation with the "Psychic Protection" exercise given later in the book.

After you practice this exercise for a short time, you will find that you can call on it quickly when you need to set a boundary, prevent energy drain, and connect with yourself. Let's say you're talking on the phone to someone, and you start to feel your energy going. You let them do the talking for a few moments, because they probably are anyway, and you close your eyes and take a deep breath. Imagine quickly that line of golden light traveling around your body, setting your boundary. Feel the energy flow through you. Open your eyes. Most likely, you'll find yourself saying, politely but firmly, whatever it is you need to say in the situation. "Let's continue this conversation another time." "OK, I'll certainly think about what you've said, but I really have to go now."

When you hang up, take another breath, redraw the line, and feel your energy. Come back. Don't stay caught in the other person's energy. Draw the line over and over, as often as you need to. If you don't have time to do it right then, do it later, at the first available moment.

Interestingly, some people tell me they feel selfish when they do this exercise, as though they don't have a right to their own energy. Or fear will arise: if I draw this line I'm separating myself; I'll end up isolated, cut off, alone. Notice what comes up for you as you try this, and know: you have a right to your personal energy. You need it. You deserve it. Focusing on yourself in this way will not isolate you, cut you off, or alienate others. It will provide a solid energetic foundation for relating to the world, your life, and other people.

Others have protested that this exercise seems negative; they don't want to see other people as threats. They prefer to love and embrace those who come their way. This exercise can be done with love—love for yourself and love for others. It is helpful for those who are highly empathic, who feel what others feel and take on the negative energies of people around them, and who tend to feel overwhelmed by other people and get lost in relationship.

The more you experiment with and reflect on the principle of conservation of energy, containment of energy, the more you will see how energy pours out of you every day. You will perhaps find yourself thinking in a different way. Rather than asking yourself in the morning, "Do I feel like doing this today?" you may ask yourself, "Will this support my energy today?" Rather than saying to yourself, "Oh, no, I can't stand this person; they drive me crazy," you might say, "This person really drains my energy; if I'm going to be with her today, I need to be extra careful to conserve and recharge my energy."

You will see how you pull the plug on yourself. You may also see ways in which you drain the energy of others. To explore the principle of conserving energy opens new windows on the world—new ways of seeing yourself and others.

Calming Your Energy

TO CALM THE ENERGY, SIMPLY CLOSE YOUR EYES, FOCUS ON YOUR BREATH, AND count the breaths. Inhale, one, exhale, two, inhale, three, and so on. Count up to ten, and back to one. You will feel the tension in the body and the mind begin to subside almost immediately. Do this for ten seconds or half an hour. Sometimes, you'll find you've counted up to thirty-five without realizing it or lost the count entirely. Just start over.

That's the simple, quick version. However, sometimes you need more. People can be overwhelmed by their own states of mind. We feel powerless, as though we are drowning in waves of thought and feeling. We need to learn how to play with all these states of mind in order to move through them with greater ease. Read through the following scenario and then experiment with it. Become the director of your own drama. You probably know quite well that your imagination can make you fearful and worried; however, your imagination can also make you calm, and when you are calm you will generally feel that you have more energy.

Riding the Waves

Imagine that you are sailing in a boat across a smooth sea. The sky is bright blue; the breeze is gentle. Everywhere there is vast, open space. You can breathe deeply. You relax.

The boat simply carries you along. Suddenly, the wind picks up, the waves get bigger, and clouds appear on the horizon. First thing you know, the boat is being tossed around like a stick, the waves are swamping you, and you are clinging to the mast for your life. The sky is dark. The wind grows even stronger and howls in your ears. The waves pound over you. You are sure you are drowning; you can barely hold on. The boat breaks apart, but you manage to keep your head above water and to grab onto a floating board.

Just as suddenly as it arose, the storm begins to subside. The wind dies down. The sea becomes calm. You relax your grip on the board and float, rocking gently on the now smooth sea. Land appears in the distance, and the current carries you toward it. You let yourself be carried right up onto the shore.

You lie there in the wet sand, feeling the earth below you and the rhythm of the waves as they wash up on the shore and recede—in and out, ebb and flow. Over and over, the waves sweep over your feet and legs and move back out; the tide goes out and out. You are on firm ground. The storm is over.

This particular scene is played out in the mind over and over. Almost every day, we experience storms, near drowning, gasping for air, fighting to stay afloat, the relief when the storm subsides, the joy of firm ground. The storm can be a fight with a partner, an interaction with a coworker, having a driver cut you off in traffic, or an item on the evening news. It can be a storm of thoughts: *What should I do? I should have done this. Why did he do this? Why doesn't she do this?* We may think we're just worrying about something, that we're just angry, or that something has just upset us a little, but our mind is experiencing a major storm. Think of how much energy it would take to go through a storm like the one described above; think of how tired you'd be afterwards, and be kind to yourself when you're tired at the end of a day of storms.

You can choose how long the storm lasts. First, become aware of how much you are tossed around by events—how a single word, a look from another person, or a passing comment can disturb your energy. Notice where in the body you feel this disturbance.

Do your jaws clench? Perhaps your solar plexus tightens or you feel queasy; perhaps your legs tense up. Find where in the body you hang on, and relax that place.

Focus on your breath. Count it. Then simply experience your breath: breathing in, breathing out, you feel the breath come and go, rise and fall.

Imagine that those waves are pounding all around you. Visualize them; feel them. Then, with a slow and wonderful exhalation, imagine them subsiding. By imagining the waves, you are bringing up into consciousness the disturbances that can actually occur in your energy when you encounter external stimuli. Once those waves are in consciousness—once you are aware of them—you can work with them. Try it. Slow them down, then make them disappear. Every time a new worry, a new tension, arises, see it as a wave. Let it subside. Or let go and be carried away. Imagine the calm of the twilight sea at low tide. Feel the shore beneath your feet. Or imagine that you are on a high cliff overlooking the storm. You can see the waves below, you can feel the wind, but you stand above the waves. Looking down, you can see them for what they are— waves that rise and fall on a vast sea.

Whatever disturbance you are experiencing, you can stand back a little and get a different perspective, without denying the experience or your feelings. You can learn to play with the storm.

Experiment for yourself. Try it now. It's good to simulate a storm, to practice this when you're not in the midst of the turbulence. Sit down; count your breaths for a few moments. Then in your imagination, create the scene of the storm and create its ending. You can visualize it, tell yourself a story, or simply sense the waves rising and quieting around you. You'll be amazed how many ways there are to bring calm to a storm. Some days, you may want to surrender and let yourself be carried away. You can be the island from which the waves are receding at low tide. Some days, you can be Moses parting the Red Sea. Or in your imagination you can even walk on water. You will find there are many ways to steer through a storm—many routes to the calm harbor, the place of peace and refuge that is always waiting in your own consciousness.

Breath as Energy

BREATH IS ENERGY. THIS SHOULD BE FAIRLY OBVIOUS. WITHOUT BREATH YOU die. Breath is the vehicle, the transmitter, of life force. Many meditative traditions work with the breath to induce altered states of consciousness, to balance the flow of energy in the body, to awaken the energy centers known as chakras, and to bring greater physical health to the body. The study of these systems can be very helpful, but a simple awareness of the breath as nourishment, as life itself, can be healing and energizing.

Many creation stories throughout the world recognize the power of breath. One Latin word for breath is "spiritus," which is also the root of the English word "spirit." Breath invests us with life. It is always with us. At any moment of the day or night, we can pay attention to our breath and experience a connection to the universal life force.

Spiritus

Simply breathe in. Notice your breath. Don't try to control it. Breathe out. Think of the breath as nourishment, as life energy. As you breathe in, feel the breath penetrate all through your body. Imagine the energy that it is carrying to each cell. Every organ is being washed by the energy of that breath, nourished by it. All you are doing in this meditation is consciously acknowledging what is happening every time you breathe.

Feel what a gift it is, this breath. So simple. A little breath brings you so much energy, every moment of every day. Perhaps a sense of wonder and appreciation arises.

You don't have to breathe any special way or do any special exercise. Every breath, just as it is, brings you life and energy. Notice the rhythm of your breathing. Notice how it changes on its own as you bring awareness to it.

The breath will serve as a vehicle for whatever energy you choose to put into it. You can breathe in colors. You can breathe in a particular word, such as *peace, abundance, joy,* or *health.* You can also breathe those qualities out into the world and send them out into the universe.

Breathing in the Insight

The breath also serves as an anchor, a way of centering and grounding yourself. It helps you to remember yourself. There is an exercise I call "Breathing in the Insight" that helps people to ground their understandings, the knowing that comes through inner work. Let's imagine you've had one of those revelations today. It seems so small, so obvious, and yet it reverberates all the way through your being. *I don't have to take care of everybody in the world,* or *I have choice,* or perhaps *I don't have to please everybody.* You know those insights. They come with such clarity, and then they disappear in the flood of daily activity, old habits, or interactions with others.

The next time such an insight comes to you, take a moment to sit down and breathe it in. Reflect on it, dwell on it, and breathe it in, deep into your body. Feel the insight, the learning, and the knowing penetrate deep into your cells. Breathe it in again, feel it become a part of you.

The breath is a tangible reminder of universal abundance. It's always there, always giving, always supporting your life. If you are seeking greater abundance in your life, receive and enjoy the gift of your breath. It's your constant companion. With awareness of your breath and the energy it brings, you are never alone.

Cleansing and Recharging Your Energy

SEVERAL YEARS AGO, I FOUND THAT MY WORK WITH PEOPLE WAS TIRING ME out and draining my energy. I began to study with teachers experienced in working with energy, Tu and Láné Moonwalker. One day as I was on my way to visit them, I saw an amazing rainbow. It was a column of color—a circular rainbow reaching from sky to earth, cloud to mountain. I have never seen anything like it. Later that day, I learned the rainbow wash, an exercise for cleansing and recharging personal energy. Here is a variation of that exercise, as it has been transformed in my work with people.

The Rainbow Wash

Imagine that you are standing or sitting under a rainbow. The rainbow moves through you from head to foot. Imagine that all the colors of the rainbow are passing through your body—red, orange, yellow, green, blue, and purple. You can visualize this, feel it, or simply tell yourself it is happening. It may pass through you in waves or one color at a time. Feel the colors pass through you and out your feet, dissolving away into white light. Ask the rainbow to cleanse your energy; ask that any negative energies expelled in this process be returned to the light.

It's good to follow this meditation with the rainbow shield, which is described in the next chapter. I learned it in conjunction with the rainbow wash.

Do this often. You can spend a long time doing it, or you can do it quickly. I do this meditation in between sessions with people, after running errands, at night before I go to sleep, and when I wake up in the morning.

As the color passes through you, it cleanses, recharges, and balances you. Don't take my word for it. Try it now.

Psychic Protection

HAVE YOU EVER FELT FATIGUED AND DRAINED SIMPLY FROM GOING TO THE grocery store? Being in a crowd of people? Does the thought of going to a class, party, lecture, or movie make you feel instantly tired? Do feelings of inexplicable sadness sometimes well up in you for no apparent reason? Do you often just want to curl up by yourself and tell the whole world to go away?

Some people are extremely empathic, which simply means they are sensitive to other people's energies and emotions. They find it hard to feel good if someone else is feeling bad; they take on the problems and worries of others. Such a person can experience simply walking down the street as a drain on his or her energy. If you are such a person, then you know how much crowds of people, or even a single unhappy or angry individual, can affect you. It's as though you have antennae out all the time, sensing the feelings and needs of others—even the person you stand behind in line at the grocery store. You notice everything. And if someone is feeling bad, you immediately feel that it's up to you to do something about it.

Many men and women are aware of this sensitivity in themselves and don't know what to do about it; they experience it as a weakness, a shortcoming. They're used to being told that they're too emotional, that they overreact, that they are too intense. People with this sensitivity may learn early to shut down their feelings out of self-protection, but empathy can't really be shut down. Misunderstood or denied, this kind of sensitivity leads to fatigue and depression. When one learns how to work with it, it can be a great gift. Empathy enhances the ability to love and understand another. It creates the desire to relate to others with kindness and compassion.

If none of the characteristics described above apply to you, you can probably skip this chapter. If you recognize yourself, consider that you may need to learn some basic techniques of psychic protection. This sounds esoteric, but it is really quite simple. Many ancient traditions teach methods of psychic protection. By this time, you have observed for yourself that your energy is affected by your interactions with the energies of other people, places, and things. Perhaps you have also begun to experience that you can use your mind to affect your energy. A basic premise of psychic protection is that you can use your mind to minimize your susceptibility to the energies of others.

The first step in psychic protection is awareness. Notice who or what drains your energy. The exercises of setting boundaries and returning energy to others are forms of psychic protection. Surrounding oneself with light is a time-honored form of psychic protection. One form of this practice is an exercise called the rainbow shield. This exercise is very simple, and it is best done after the rainbow wash.

The Rainbow Shield

Every morning before you leave your house, do the rainbow wash exercise, and then imagine yourself surrounded by rainbow light. You can imagine the spectrum of light with red closest to your body, or purple—whatever feels right to you. The colors in the rainbow go from red to orange, then yellow, green, blue, and purple. The rainbow extends out in every direction from your body as far as you would like. It can be a sphere, or it can shape itself to your body as an aura. You can visualize this or simply tell yourself that it is there.

Return to your awareness of this rainbow light throughout the day, especially if you are feeling tired. Practice the rainbow wash again as you fall asleep, and imagine the shield around you as you fall asleep.

This works. I don't know how. I can't explain it logically. But if you find yourself drained by people and events in your life, try it regularly for a while. See what happens.

This psychic protection exercise calls you back to yourself. One of the main ways we lose energy to people is by focusing on them, obsessing over them, and forgetting ourselves. The next time you find yourself in a difficult situation and you're alone, thinking about it, and trying to figure out what to do, don't spend hours going over what happened, what might happen, or what you should have said or shouldn't have. Don't beat yourself up. Come back to the rainbow shield. Feel yourself in the middle of that rainbow light; return to yourself. Yes, you will have to deal with the situation, but for the moment, retreat into this peaceful, protected space you have learned to create for yourself. Restore your energy. From this place, you will be better able to see your course of action clearly.

Reclaiming Your Energy

··

THE TIBETAN BUDDHISTS HAVE MANY TEACHINGS THAT VIVIDLY DESCRIBE the *bardo*, the state the consciousness experiences after death. According to their beliefs, the consciousness travels through the bardo, experiencing many colors of light, many fearsome experiences, many beautiful ones, encountering deities and demons, being pulled this way and that by powerful forces, until finally it is reborn in a new physical form. The classic *Tibetan Book of the Dead* describes these forces vividly as having the power of a tornado.[4] Many of the practices of Tibetan Buddhism are intended to help one traverse the bardo, staying focused in awareness and not being overwhelmed by the powerful karmic forces of greed, anger, and ignorance, so that one can be reborn in a state of love and awareness.

Regardless of whether you believe in reincarnation and the Tibetan view of what happens after death, the image of the bardo is a powerful metaphor for our journey through this world, in life as well as in death. Every day we experience the pulls and forces of old habits and patterns. We see ourselves doing the same old things over and over, and we keep doing them. The patterns repeat themselves. We make up our minds to go one way, and we end up going another. We resolve to do this or that, and the days, months, years slip away. The Tibetans teach that we must learn not to be deceived by appearances. What we encounter in the bardo may appear to be beautiful, but underneath it may be destructive. Or we may meet a wrathful deity that appears terrible but in fact may wish to help us. We get pulled by appearances all the time; we go through life being attracted to this or that experience, person, place, group, cause, spiritual path, teacher, teaching, belief system, and so on. Often, we end up losing our energy to whatever it is we have been attracted to. We lose ourselves in the appearance—in the belief that this person, place, or thing holds love, truth, and salvation.

No matter how much you do the exercise of conserving energy, you will still find yourself in situations that pull on your energy. It's part of the human experience. You'll still sometimes feel overwhelmed by people or events. Undoubtedly in your life you've already lost some of your energy to people—parents, partners, teachers, bosses, or friends. As you work with containing and conserving your energy, you'll become more skilled at recognizing when your energy has been drained and when you need to reclaim it. You may realize how little energy you habitually save for yourself. You get better at guiding yourself through the bardo of this life with its terrible and beautiful experiences, its sorrows and joys. You get better at saying, "Here I choose to give of myself, to share and exchange my energy; here, I choose to detach, to draw in my energy, to reclaim it."

Read through this exercise first and then try it for yourself.

Reclamation

Think now of a person in your life, past or present, who has taken energy from you or overwhelmed you. It's better to start with someone who is just an average energy drain—perhaps someone you work with, a teacher if you're in school, or a longtime friend whose boundaries aren't so great. You can work up to those deep old energy drains—a self-involved parent who demanded your very life energy to feed and support his or her own, a close friend or partner who betrayed you, a spiritual teacher who misused power, or any one of many possibilities. This exercise can help to heal those deep, old wounds that still bleed energy, but this work may best be done with the presence and support of a friend or healer.

Draw the line of light around yourself. Feel your border, your boundary, and your energy moving through you. Spend some time there with yourself. Then visualize or think of the other person.

Notice what happens as you do this. As soon as you think of the other person, you'll experience a reaction in your energy. What is it? Is it an emotional one—fear or anger or grief? Is it a physical sensation? Some people experience a literal pull, as though the person were a magnet. You may lose the line around you. You may feel energy pouring out of you, perhaps through the solar plexus. Just notice your reaction. Be with it for a while.

Come back to yourself, draw the line of light, take a breath, and feel your energy. Practice bringing the person present in your mind and making her go away. If you visualize easily, you can close your eyes, see the person appear, and then see him recede into a cloud of golden light. Otherwise, you can simply imagine this or sense it. Tell yourself it is happening: "The image of X is receding into the light."

Experiment with describing the person by a label rather than a name: "the coworker" or "the teacher." See if that approach reduces or increases the energy reaction. Don't be discouraged if you have hard time imagining the person receding into the light. Just keep practicing it.

Next, think of the person, notice your reaction, draw the line of light around yourself, and imagine that your energy goes out to this person like a wave. Let yourself feel the pull. Then, slowly, carefully, imagine that you are reeling your energy back in, just as if you were a fisherman pulling in a fish. Carefully and patiently imagine your energy returning to you. Draw it right into your solar plexus. Feel it come back to you as warmth and light. Let it enter you; feel it circulate through you. Imagine the person receding into the light and being surrounded by light.

You don't necessarily have to feel good and kind and loving toward the person. You can still be angry, fearful, or tense. Perhaps after this experience you can be more neutral. This exercise is not about changing how you feel about this person, although it may have that effect. It's about helping you detach your energy from theirs. The important thing is that over and over, you return your attention to your own energy—to drawing it back, receiving it into you, and feeling it fill you.

If when you finish, you are still disturbed by the other's presence, know that using this technique takes practice. Be patient and give it time. If just imagining the presence of that person disturbs your energy so much, think what the actual presence of the person does! So if you keep working with this, chances are you'll get better at reclaiming your energy and detaching it from this person. Eventually, you will be able to do it in the actual presence of the person. This exercise can be done with situations, events, groups of people, and even places.

Many Buddhist meditations focus on developing both compassion and detachment in relation to others. These may seem to be contradictory attitudes, but in fact, compassion flows much more easily in the presence of detachment. As you learn to reclaim your energy, to literally "un-attach" it from the energy of another, you won't necessarily come to like that person more, but you may find yourself feeling greater compassion and being more able to see where the person is coming from. You may be able to send the person this energetic message: "I wish you well, even as I choose not to get involved with your energy." As you pay attention to your energy, becoming sensitive to its ups and downs in a new way, you may also feel greater compassion for yourself, a natural desire to take care of yourself.

Compassion and detachment are two habits of mind that help us to find our way through our bardo of the moment. Most people I meet are deeply compassionate. They feel the suffering of others and are acutely aware of the world's pain. Detachment, however, is often a foreign concept to them. Working with the energy of detachment balances this intense compassion and gives you firmer ground to stand on in this world.

None of these exercises have to be followed to the letter. Read them through, try them out, and see where they take you. You will find that even as you simply read them, they are already happening at some level. You may even find that just by reading the exercises, you have more energy! Energy is mysterious and wonderful. The possibilities are infinite.

Returning Energy
to Others

IN THE JAPANESE MARTIAL ART OF AIKIDO, PEOPLE ARE TAUGHT TO DEFEND themselves by returning the energy of an attack. One's intent in this martial art is not to harm, to win, or to overpower, but rather to protect oneself by flowing with the energy. Simply by stepping out of the way at the right moment, one can neutralize an attack.

This concept can be applied in many circumstances. We all experience emotional or mental attacks at times. Sometimes, they're intentional: another person overtly abuses, hurts, or betrays us. Sometimes, other people simply are carrying so much negative energy that they're throwing it off randomly; we take it in and experience it as an attack or invasion. Sensitive people will often learn as children to unconsciously take on the negative energy of others; a child will absorb and carry a parent's unconscious grief, fear, or anger. This creates a weight in one's energy; people may actually feel a heaviness that they have carried all their lives but can't identify. So it's important to learn how to return negative energy to others and how to not take it on in the first place.

Stepping Aside

Let's begin with a simple situation. You're on the phone with your father, mother, sister, neighbor, or boss. You pick the person. We'll call him or her X. X is going on and on about something. You pick the situation. In the course of the conversation, during which X is doing most of the talking, you begin to feel tired. X is fearful, angry, or worried. You become aware that you are supposed to do something about this. You're trying. You're listening and you're making a suggestion here and there, but you know you're not getting through.

Disengage your mind from the conversation, take a breath, yes, draw that line of light (standard procedure by now), and think: *This is your anger (grief, fear, pain), not mine. I return it to you, with the prayer that you may find help and light and strength to deal with it. I will help you in any way I can, but this is your energy, not mine.*

Imagine the person surrounded by a golden light. If the person has a particular religion or spiritual path, imagine a saint or deity, helper or teacher from that path being with the person, helping them. Or imagine a line of golden light connecting them to a great cloud of golden light that represents their connection to the universal source. In doing this, you are not simply sending the energy back, you are adding a prayer for healing. Return to the conversation, but disengage from it as often as necessary.

This exercise is really simple, but it's amazing how often people will feel guilty about doing it, as though they are going to harm the other person by returning the energy, or as though it's their responsibility to take on the negative energy. You can help people much more effectively if you don't take on their energy—if you remember there are greater healing powers in the universe that can also help them. It's not all up to you.

This is just a beginning. Applying this principle is complex and requires endless creativity. It takes a lot of training from a qualified teacher and a high degree of skill to apply it if you are being physically attacked. At the level of energy, however, you can begin by simply reflecting on this fact: in many situations that arise in interactions with people, you have a choice. You don't have to take on the negative energy of other people or external situations.

There is a completely different way of returning energy to others, based on a meditation practice in Tibetan Buddhism called *tonglen.* In this practice, one consciously chooses to absorb and transform the negativity and suffering of others.

Tonglen

Here is a simple version of this practice: Sit quietly, following the breath and calming the mind. Imagine the negativity of the world, or a particular person or situation, as a dark cloud. Breathe it in, draw it down into your heart, and imagine that it is transformed into light. Feel it be transformed, the weight dissolve, and the dark lighten. Breathe the light back out into the world with the wish that it travel far, for the good of all beings.

The excellent book *Start Where You Are*, by Pema Chodron, offers detailed guidance in tonglen practice.[5]

The tonglen meditation is a good one to do when you experience that particular energy drain that comes from feeling disempowered in the face of war, oppression, or injustice. When you feel helpless in the presence of global suffering, don't try to deny it. Sit down, breathe it in, transform it, and breathe out compassion and light. Then see how you can actualize that practice in the world, in ways large and small.

If one approach encourages you to return negative energy to its source, then why consciously choose to take it on? How does that help? There is a big difference between consciously taking in negativity for the purpose of transforming it and unconsciously absorbing and carrying negative energies. What matters is having a lot of tools to choose from. What works for you? What helps you to resolve a problem with a particular person? What helps you to feel more peaceful? You may need to learn you have a right to say no to another's negative energies. You may need to feel your power to transform negative energy. It's not a matter of a right way or a wrong way to work with energy—a higher or a lower path. It's about being creative, flexible, and energetic in your responses to the situations that arise in your life. It's about not being overpowered by them.

Releasing Energy Through Choice

....

I have choice.

Affirm this to yourself over and over again—morning, noon, and night. To recognize that you have choice and to accept the responsibility of exercising choice gives you enormous energy. It addresses deep old feelings of powerlessness. Low energy is associated with a feeling of powerlessness. The more you experience your power of choice, the more energy you will have.

Often, our conditioning teaches us we have no choice. Exercise and be aware of your power of choice whenever possible. You choose what you eat for breakfast, what route you take to work, what you do in the evening. Become aware of how much choice you have. Notice your choices.

Many people in the world don't have much choice and haven't throughout human history. Most of us carry the collective unconscious experience of powerlessness. For centuries, people's lives were defined for them: their roles in society, their life partners, their religions, and their values were chosen for them by society and the family. Now, many of the institutions that used to define human lives are crumbling. We have to choose our partners, professions, religions, and values. People often retreat from these choices. They say, "I don't know what I should do," or "I don't know what my purpose is."

People often continue to react to external situations as though they were still children, or slaves, or soldiers, citizens from an ancient time when strict rules dictated their lives.

They look for commands to obey, rules to follow, instructions, and answers, even when their present lives have few such restrictions. Notice what comes up when you think, *I have choice.* Often, the first reaction is *I don't want choice. I hate making decisions.* If you are really honest, you may feel you wish you didn't have choice—that someone would just make your decisions for you.

Acknowledging this response if it occurs is important. Explore it. Do you really wish that? Even though choice is difficult and demanding—even though it requires a willingness to risk, self-knowledge, and letting go of control, because you can't know what will happen—wouldn't you rather have a choice than have a parent, government, or religious institution tell you what to do?

The awareness *I have choice* and the commitment to choosing choice rather than avoiding it is a crucial growing-up point in the individual and the global human consciousness. The tendency to blame and project, to look for both scapegoats and saviors, is a common human experience.

It is helpful to realize that you make your choices within a framework—on the basis of your life experiences, values, and belief systems. Spend a day reflecting on your values, spiritual aspirations, beliefs, and goals in life. State them clearly to yourself, in writing if you choose. Don't accept the inner voice that might say, "I don't know what my purpose is. I don't know why I'm here." You do know why you're here and what you think life is about for you. Affirm that you know this, and let it emerge from deep inside you, your deep feelings of what you want from this life, what you want to learn and experience.

Do you want to love, learn, heal, grow, and be of service? Do you want to express your inner self? Find meaningful work? Have children? Do you want to devote your life to seeking God? Do you want to be a musician, a lawyer, an actor, or a cook? Do you want to enjoy your life? Help the planet? None of the above? Do you want to climb mountains? Learn to relax? The possibilities are endless. Do you want to experience life in its fullness? To find meaning and joy? Do you want to travel, do research, or invent something new? Do you want to experience comfort, ease, and warmth? Do you want to make a lot of money? Do you want to help those who are suffering? Do you want to learn to communicate better and help others to do so? Do you want to experience health and well-being? Do you want even more—something so unique and personal to yourself it can't be imagined by another? Don't judge your desires. Let them be.

Use them as a basis from which to make your choices from day to day. Ask yourself if the choice you're making, whether large or small, supports your vision and your aspirations.

You can release a lot of energy by recognizing that you have choice about your inner state and how you respond to external circumstances. You can choose how you think, feel, and respond to any given situation. Your inner response does not have to be dictated by external circumstances. In realizing this, you begin to truly create your own reality.

For example, perhaps you know someone who always makes you angry. What are your choices? The person may be irritating, but only you can become irritated. How can you change your response? The next time you meet the person, begin by standing back energetically, drawing that line of light around yourself, and reminding yourself, *I have choice about how I respond to this person.* This doesn't mean you have to be nice and loving. You can reclaim your energy, return the energy to the person, or look at what you need to communicate. There are countless possibilities.

Many people feel overwhelmed by their own internal states. Their feelings are so strong they cannot find themselves in the midst of the waves of emotion—the overpowering depression, guilt, anxiety, or anger. Some of the methods described in this book can provide a raft in the storm, something to hold on to while you ride out the waves of strong emotion, or a path through the confusing complexity of our human feelings. The meditations in the chapters on "Calming Your Energy," "Releasing the Energy Caught in Old Psychological Patterns," and "Awareness as Energy" can all give you greater choice about how to respond to your inner emotional states. These practices can help prevent you from being overwhelmed by your own mind and losing energy. You don't even have to do the exercises. Just pick up the book, open it to "Calming Your Energy," and read it over and over until you feel like doing it. Then do it.

The brief affirmation, the constant reminder *I have choice*, is one of the most important things you can do to increase your energy. Try it. Breathe quietly. Allow the words *I have choice* to penetrate your consciousness. Breathe the words *I have choice* through your whole body.

Making choice also means developing your intuition, including your ability to sense what is right for you. It means trusting your inner knowing. Our conditioning does not encourage this. People get caught in wheels of obsessive thought when they have to make choices; they keep trying to figure it out.

When you are making a choice, you may need to consult the chapter "Thought as Energy." It may be necessary to dissolve away some obsessive thought patterns and let go of some worries before you can see and feel clearly.

Here is an exercise that can help you feel your choices more tangibly in any given situation. It will bring you greater awareness—and intuition is awareness, a knowing that comes from beyond the rational mind, from beyond your feelings, from your deep self. Use it in the context of an actual choice or decision you have to make.

Choice

Sit down and breathe quietly. Follow your breath and enter a meditative state, simply paying attention to the breath, noticing what your mind is doing but not trying to control it. Spend a few minutes in awareness meditation, noting the sensations in your body and the thoughts in your mind.

Set an intention: ask for greater awareness about this choice.

Place your hands on your knees, palms up. Become aware of your breath and the central column of the body—the spine, chest, and pelvis. Center your attention there and feel yourself from the top of your head down to the pelvis. Let the breath and the central column of the body represent you—the wholeness of yourself, the awareness in you that perceives, understands, and chooses.

Now take two alternatives. Let's use a simple example: should I go out this evening or stay home? Place one choice in one hand (it doesn't matter which one) and the other choice in the other hand.

Bring your awareness to one hand. Bring it to that choice. Feel yourself holding that choice, and then enter into it. Use your imagination. What does that alternative feel like? Imagine yourself taking that path. Feel what it feels like in your body, in your imagination. Don't think about it, but note any thoughts, questions, or insights that arise.

Withdraw your attention from the one hand and return to the breath, the central awareness. Move into the other hand. Experience that choice. Don't try to arrive at a decision. Just experience the possibilities.

Withdraw your attention from that hand and return to the central breathing awareness that is the essential you. Know that you contain all possibilities and that you can choose. Remain in that state of awareness, simply holding the choice in consciousness. Perhaps it becomes clear; perhaps you still don't know. Let it be. It will become clear.

If you like, you can bring your hands together in front of your heart. Feel the possibilities come together. Ask that whatever you choose be for your greatest good.

This exercise can also be used to experience your power of choice in relation to your inner state. Perhaps you are feeling overwhelmed by grief, fear, or anger. Reflect for a moment. What could you choose to feel instead? Joy, peace, acceptance, detachment, love for yourself?

Follow the same steps. Place one feeling in one hand and another in the other hand; for example, anger and acceptance, sorrow and joy, attachment and letting go, fear and love.

Breathe quietly and go in and out of the feelings. Remember a time you felt love, joy, acceptance, or letting go. Use that memory to reenter that feeling. Return always to the breath, the central awareness. Notice how it feels to move in and out of the feelings, and notice where you get caught. Experience the self—the loving awareness that holds all these feelings in yourself, that experiences both joy and sorrow, that is larger than anger or serenity, that is always with you.

Many people ask what they can do about the state of the world today. There is at least one simple answer: in your own life, from moment to moment, recognize your choices, honor your power of choice, consider carefully the consequences of your choices, and accept responsibility for your choices. The more people on the planet who are doing these things, the better off the planet will be.

Awareness as Energy

....

IN THE POPULAR MOVIE *GROUNDHOG DAY*, THE HERO FINDS HIMSELF LIVING the same day over and over again—until he gets it right. In one scene, he is walking down the street, wrapped up in his own thoughts. He trips over a hole in the sidewalk. The next day, which is the same day repeating itself, he trips over the hole again. We know he knows it's there. We watch him do it time after time. The fourth or fifth time through the day, he finally gets it right. He steps around the hole.

We spend a lot of energy falling into old, familiar holes and climbing out again. It seems almost impossible to see them coming and step around them. Sometimes, we spend years in one and then climb out, only to fall right back in. This falling into holes, getting stuck, and climbing out takes a lot of energy. That's why developing awareness is such an important factor in conserving and using energy.

Awareness is that in us which knows, thinks, feels, perceives, remembers, chooses, daydreams, feels, and senses. Traditionally, Western thought has located this awareness in the brain, but modern scientists are discovering what many ancient cultures knew all along: that there is an awareness that pervades the human body and indeed all sentient life. Our cells respond to visualization; prayers and music influence the growth of plants. Modern physicists theorize that phenomena at the subatomic level come into being only when they are observed. Many psychologists and anthropologists have acknowledged the power of observation: the very act of observation changes the phenomena being observed. As we begin to observe ourselves, we begin to change. Something new comes into being. Lynne McTaggart's book *The Field: The Quest for the Secret Force of the Universe* gives fascinating details of ongoing scientific research into energy and consciousness.[6]

We have an abundance of awareness available to us. The capacity of the human mind to perceive, synthesize, understand, and create is truly awesome. We don't have to develop awareness; we simply have to access it. Meditation is a doorway into a greater awareness. You can invite that awareness to come to you, to be present in your life. To name something calls its energy present; this is the principle behind the ancient practice of invocation. We begin this next meditative exercise by invoking awareness.

Awareness Meditation

As you begin this awareness meditation, sit down quietly in any comfortable posture. Say out loud whatever words you choose to invoke awareness: "I now invite the presence of awareness to come to me." "I ask to experience greater awareness in my life and in my relationships with people." Use the words that feel right to you. Say them out loud. Breathe deeply for a few moments, and then allow the breath to settle into a normal rhythm. Become aware of yourself.

Begin by experiencing the breath moving in and out of the nostrils. Feel it. Identify it. Think to yourself, *Breathing.* Become aware of your mind noticing the breath. *Noticing.* Allow the mind to travel through the body, noticing any sensations in any part of the body. Identify them. *Itching. Pain. Tension.* Notice the mind noticing the sensation. If the attention wanders, and you begin to daydream or become involved in thoughts of past or future, simply note it. *Daydreaming. Planning.*

Don't force your mind back to attention; it will naturally wander off and naturally return. Note the movement of the mind in and out of many states of emotion, reaction, and judgment. Notice that no matter how you resolve to pay attention, you find yourself in some world of fantasy, thought, or feeling. This is the nature of the mind. By practicing attention, you become more conscious of what is always happening in your mind.

This practice also develops your power of choice. Over and over, you choose to come back to a place of awareness.

Notice how your field of awareness widens and becomes more sensitive. You are simultaneously aware of sounds outside, sensations in the body, and thoughts in the mind. You are aware of being aware. This meditation opens the doorway into yourself and the vast universe that exists within you.

Practice this meditation for as long as you like, quietly breathing in and out. It can be done for a certain amount of time every day, or for a few minutes here and there throughout your day.

Often, people actually lose energy through meditation because they develop a tense relationship with it. Don't force yourself. This meditation can give you a huge amount of energy if you stop for a couple of minutes at a time regularly during the day, close your eyes briefly, and connect with your awareness.

This basic meditation described above, which comes from the vipassana, or insight, practice of Theravada Buddhism, can also carry you into another level of awareness meditation, that of self-inquiry. This is a practice in many spiritual traditions. As you meditate and experience an expanded awareness, the question "Who is it that is experiencing all of this?" will quite naturally arise. It is a great mystery. Who am I? What is it that thinks, feels, perceives, and hears? As one sits with those questions, one's sense of oneself begins to expand. Spaciousness arises in the mind. You begin to see that whatever you are, it is more than thoughts, feelings, bodily sensations, hopes and fears, likes and dislikes. You are this spacious awareness.

That spaciousness is another key to having more energy. Many people these days feel crowded—by other people, the demands of their lives, and their own inner state. Self-inquiry allows one to detach for a time from all these elements of one's life and dwell in a greater space, the space of awareness.

This practice of self-inquiry challenges our fundamental notion of self. We lose a lot of energy in self-consciousness, wondering what others are thinking of us, comparing ourselves, and judging ourselves. To question the fundamental concept of what this self is, to explore it from many perspectives, begins to loosen the tightly held habits of self-judgment. It is important in this meditation of self-inquiry that you do not try to arrive at an answer.

Self-Inquiry

Simply sit quietly, follow the breath, note the sensations, and then allow the attention to shift from the sensations to the questions: *Who am I? Am I this personality, this body, this collection of experiences? Am I my mind, my consciousness, my past, my future? Am I my thoughts and feelings? Am I what I do? Am I spirit, God, soul?* You will find your own pathways into and through these questions. They will grow and expand, mirror and reflect you to yourself, and guide you deeper into yourself. A great energy comes from this exploration—a freedom and a peace—as long as you don't look for an answer!

In the exploration itself, many insights arise that will give you energy. Trying to find "the" answer will frustrate you. The self is not one thing with one final definition. We also lose a lot of energy by trying to be some one thing. The more you explore the self, the more you will discover it to be multidimensional, constantly changing, inconsistent, beautifully unlimited in its variations, moods, thoughts, and feelings.

End this meditation with the thought *I honor this self.* Breathe that thought deep into your body, your heart. Feel the energy of that honoring nourish you through and through.

In today's world, we have a huge capacity to deny our feelings and experiences. It is a defense mechanism that comes from living in an overwhelming world, full of painful experiences, confusion, and dysfunction. Many of us learn to dissociate early in life—in our families, schools, and jobs. We often don't even know we're low on energy until we get sick. Then we say, "Well, I guess my body is trying to tell me something." Meditation is a good way to listen to yourself and get the messages before they become urgent and painful. The simple awareness meditation described above connects you with yourself. The practice of self-assessment on a regular basis can also bring you greater awareness and help you listen to yourself.

Self-Assessment

After a few moments of experiencing your breath and entering a greater awareness, check in with yourself. How am I doing, mentally, physically, emotionally, and spiritually?

Rate your energy in each of those areas, on a scale of one to ten, with ten being full of flowing energy and one being completely drained and exhausted. Am I feeling mentally positive or fatigued and overwhelmed by negative thoughts? Am I physically tired or tense, or is there a basic sense of energy, health, and well-being? At the physical level, you can become more detailed and check out specific parts of the body—the different systems, such as the digestive, reproductive, circulatory, and other systems. You can check with different organs. You will be surprised how directly your body will communicate with you!

As you pay attention in this way, you may already find your energy beginning to rise, or you may feel even more tired as you become aware of how tired you really are. Please note that the inventory is not making you more tired; it is simply putting you in touch with yourself.

Check in with your emotions: What have you recently been feeling or what are you feeling at this moment? And how is your spiritual energy? Is it flowing? Do you feel your connection with spirit, with a consciousness greater than yourself, in whatever form you experience that?

It is much harder to avoid taking care of yourself if you are assessing yourself regularly in this way. It's another way of honoring yourself. It's a practical way of loving yourself. People are often advised to love themselves, and they haven't a clue how to begin to do it. Checking in regularly with the many different aspects of yourself is a beginning. It's being courteous to yourself. With this self-assessment, you have the opportunity to ask yourself how you are and to listen to the response.

Thought as Energy

....

YOUR THOUGHTS CAN GIVE YOU MORE ENERGY, OR THEY CAN TAKE YOUR energy away.

As you did in the "you are energy" exercise, imagine that you are simply energy. Close your eyes and feel the flow and dance of that energy. Imagine everything solid around you pulsing and vibrating with energy. Think to yourself, *I am pure energy.*

If you think this often enough, you will begin to experience yourself this way. If you think, *I have no energy*, then you will experience that. It is impossible to have no energy. Remember, you can't have energy, or not have it. You are energy, and you are surrounded by it. If you think, *I am energy. Everything is energy. I am supported by all the energy in the universe*, chances are you will feel more energy. Try it. Next time you are feeling tired, stressed, and overwhelmed, don't think, *I can't stand this. I'm so tired. I never have any time. I never have enough energy.* Try thinking like this: *I'm so tired. I have so much to do. I need to take a few minutes to sit down and remember that I am energy, that everything is energy. I need to take a few minutes to breathe quietly, remembering that every breath is energy.*

In some esoteric teachings, it is said that the entire universe is created from the alphabet. The letters of the alphabet come together to form words; words then shape and define our reality. As it says in the book of Genesis, "In the beginning was the Word."

Our words—the labels we place upon our experience—to a large extent create and define our world. Therefore, it's useful to spend a day noticing your patterns of thought. What thoughts give you energy? What thoughts make you feel tired and depressed and cause you to lose energy?

Identify at least three ways that you waste or lose energy through your thoughts. Perhaps you get involved in obsessive thoughts about what you have to do. Perhaps you spend a lot of time thinking about what others think of you. Perhaps you judge yourself frequently. Notice the specific thoughts and thought patterns that repeat themselves and drain your energy. Write them down.

Can you transform energy-draining thoughts into energy-producing ones? There are many ways to change habitual thought patterns. Transforming your way of thinking is different from trying to think positively, as people are often encouraged to do. Sometimes, the attempt to impose a positive thought on a strong negative thought pattern results only in a feeling of frustration and powerlessness.

The following exercise is based on meditations from the Buddhist tradition. Buddhism teaches that all thoughts—and indeed all phenomena—have three phases: arising, staying, and dissolving. Everything arises at a certain point in time, stays for a while, and then ceases, dissolves away. Ordinarily in Buddhist practice, one simply watches the arising, the staying, and the dissolving of each thought. This exercise allows you to work actively to dissolve negative thought patterns.

Dissolution

Sit quietly and meditate with a thought pattern you've identified that repeats itself again and again. Crystallize it into a few simple words. Get the essence of it: *I can't.* Keep it short: *I'll never be good enough.* And so on. Visualize the words floating in a field of golden light, as though they are on a movie screen at a distance from you. Let the words dissolve one by one into the light. Bring the statement back and dissolve it letter by letter. Each letter dissolves away into golden light. Again, you can either active-ly visualize this process or tell yourself it is happening, word-by-word, letter-by-letter, or you can both visualize and verbalize the process. This practice takes time and patience. You might even get bored, which means the thought is already losing its power. You might decide there are a lot of other things you'd rather be doing than messing around with this particular thought. Great! Go do some of them!

Meditation is a creative process. You will discover many ways to free your mind of its old patterns and thereby release your energy. You can find an image for the thought pattern. For example, many people see obsessive thinking as a hamster running around on a wheel. Spend some time with the image. Explore it. See it at a distance, as on a movie screen again. Dissolve it away into the light.

Perhaps as you dissolve away a thought, you become aware of a particular emotion beneath it: fear, anger, or guilt, for example. As you spend time with the feeling, you may be able to trace the thought pattern back to its childhood root, to see how you learned to think this way.

As you explore a thought in this way, as you stay with the process, breathing quietly, and then dissolve the thought away into the light, you may experience that there then is only energy. You can experience the energy at the root of the thought and understand how much energy goes into the creation and maintenance of these complex thought patterns. Even if you just for one moment experience a space between the thoughts—a moment of pure energy, the dissolution of the thought—in that one moment you are in touch with a universal energy, that life force energy of creation before "the word."

Two of the most common negative thought patterns are worry and obsessive thinking. When you find these patterns draining your energy, these two simple approaches may work for you.

When you find yourself worrying, first simply acknowledge that you can't help it. You want things to go well; you want your friends or loved ones to be well. You worry about them, or the future, or the world, or any of a number of other things. See if you can shift the energy into prayer. A worried thought arises. Become aware of it; identify it. Think, *Okay. I'm worrying.* Take a breath, notice what's happening to your energy as you worry, and see if you can say a prayer instead. Pray to whomever or whatever you regard as the greater power. Pray for help, the greatest good, or a specific outcome. If you're worried about others, say a prayer, light a candle for them, and surround them with light. Some of the oldest, simplest rituals in human experience are remarkably effective.

All negative thought patterns tend to be repetitive. That's what makes them so energy-draining. A thought comes up, you talk yourself out of it, feel better briefly, and there it is again. The obsessive quality of negative thought patterns creates a feeling of powerlessness, which in turn leads to a feeling of low energy.

Using a mantra is a time-honored spiritual practice that is effective in shifting the energy around obsessive thinking. Traditionally, a mantra is a sacred sound, word, or divine name. It is repeated over and over. The purpose of repeating a mantra is not only to calm the mind but also to attune the mind to a vibration of peace and love. Obsessive thinking is like a musical instrument out of tune; a mantra helps to bring the mind into harmony. In obsessive thinking, the mind is repeating a thought over and over; it clearly has the power to repeat a thought. Why not let it repeat a thought that will create harmony rather than further discord?

There are hundreds of mantras. Traditionally it is said that to be effective, a mantra is best received from a spiritual teacher. For certain purposes of meditation, this is so. However, if you don't have access to such a teacher, and you want to use a mantra to calm the mind, to shift your energy, and to free the mind from habitual thought patterns, experiment for yourself. Choose a mantra, or more than one, that feels right to you—that brings a sense of peace and harmony. Then say it, think it, over and over. The mind will take it up; it becomes like an underlying rhythm in your consciousness. You can shift your attention to it more and more easily when negative thought patterns arise. The mantra steadies the mind and gives it a focus other than the habitual thought pattern.

One common mantra is simply "Om." In the Hindu tradition, this is considered to be the most sacred sound, a sound that contains the whole universe. It is the word of creation.

Mantras are often simply divine names repeated over and over: Jesus Christ; Mary, Mother of God; Tara; Rama; Allah; God. In the Tibetan tradition, the mantra "Om Mani Padme Hum" attunes the consciousness to a state of serenity and compassion. A great mantra of the Hindu tradition is "Om Nama Shivaya," which honors the Divine in all of us. The Christian mantra "Maranatha" comes from the ancient Aramaic and means "Come Lord."[7] The Buddhist prayer "May all beings be happy, peaceful, and free of suffering" is a wonderful one because it shifts one's energy from concern with one's personal problems to the larger picture. A word such as peace, love, joy, abundance, or harmony can become a mantra. The book *Healing Mantras*, by Thomas Ashley-Farrand, offers expert guidance in mantra practice from the Eastern spiritual traditions,[8] and *Word into Silence*, by John Main, gives instructions for the use of mantra in a Christian context.[9]

These exercises are not about getting rid of thoughts, which is sometimes considered to be a goal of meditation. The mind makes thoughts; that's its nature. As you continue to develop your awareness, you will discover that you have the ability to choose the thoughts the mind thinks and to slow down the pace or speed it up. The awareness is the musician; the mind is the instrument. It can be tuned to play a different melody.

To transform one's thinking takes ongoing patience and commitment to oneself. It's another way of practicing love for yourself. You give attention to yourself when you pay attention to your thought processes—when you tune the instrument of your mind. It's a day-to-day, moment-to-moment process. Don't be discouraged if negative thought patterns continue to arise. Musical instruments need continual tuning; no musician would think it possible to tune an instrument only once or twice and have it stay in tune. This constant attention sometimes takes serious effort. Sometimes it's fun, a game to play with yourself.

If you think of your mind as an enemy and try to fight it, you'll probably lose. If you treat your mind like a misbehaving child and scold it, it will rebel. The exercises in this chapter are about making friends with your mind, getting to know your thought patterns, exploring them, and playing with them.

Releasing Energy Stuck in Old Belief Systems

....

WHAT IS A BELIEF SYSTEM? IT'S A PATTERN IN CONSCIOUSNESS, A STRUCTURE IN the psyche. It's an attitude towards life you have learned. We inherit our belief systems from our culture, our experience, and our ancestors. Belief systems organize our lives; they determine our behavior and how we think. They are simplistic, black and white, and cast in stone. You can't argue with a belief system. It's always right. That's its defining characteristic. You can't communicate with a belief system. You can't convince it. It doesn't listen. It doesn't recognize shades and hues of different perspectives and possibilities. No matter how hard you work, how you try to convince yourself you don't *really* believe that, the belief system sits there in your consciousness like a rock.

Here are some common belief systems one encounters over and over in the contemporary human consciousness:

I'm bad.

There's something wrong with me.

No one listens to me.

No matter what I do, I always mess it up.

If I really love someone, I'll get hurt.

No one loves me. (Variation: No one will ever love me.)

Men want to control me (if you're a woman).

Women want to control me (if you're a man).

I can't.

I have to be good (nice) or no one will love me.

Everybody leaves me.

I can either be creative and fulfilled or I can be responsible, but not both.

Anger is bad.

Nothing matters.

Nothing I do matters.

I can be spiritual or worldly, but not both.

These are but a few of the belief systems that people hold. I call them systems because no one belief arises alone. "I'm bad" is connected to "Everyone leaves me," which returns to "I'm bad" and then connects again to "I can't." These beliefs are based on experience and conditioning. It's hard to affirm what isn't in your experience. It's hard to convince yourself that people do listen to you, or might, when your past experience is that they don't.

You may well have beautiful and positive, life-affirming belief systems. We will look at ways to help these beliefs give you more energy, but for now we're talking about the ones that get in the way.

The energy of a belief system is dense and heavy; it bears the weight of accumulated experience. This heaviness is not metaphorical; you will experience it when you begin to work with your belief systems. Working energetically with a belief system can be powerful; you're no longer trying to fight it, trying to not believe it, wishing it would go away, being frustrated by it. You are bringing the light of your awareness to it and allowing that light to penetrate the old, dense structure.

Working with Belief Systems

The first step in working with belief systems, as in working with your thoughts, is to identify some of your most basic beliefs. Sit down quietly, pay attention to the breath, draw a line of light around yourself, and ask yourself, "What do I believe, deep inside myself, about myself, life, relationship, work, people, the world, the universe?" Begin with yourself. What do you believe about yourself? Whatever emerges, try to keep it in short, simple, black-and-white terms. Don't get into a long discussion with yourself about how you don't really believe this, or about how sometimes you do and sometimes you don't. Admit it: I believe this.

This admission—this surrender to your deepest belief systems—is a very important step. Experience a sense of wonder: "Wow, I really believe this. This is what runs me." If you let yourself see that you really hold a belief, you will immediately understand much more about your habitual patterns of behavior. Usually, people try to deny their deep beliefs about themselves or the world because they're afraid of them. They don't want to believe they really believe that.

Once you've identified a belief system and surrendered to it, feel it all the way through your body. Don't be discouraged. Once a belief is up in consciousness—once you've identified it in its most blatant form and admitted you believe in it—it's already lost some of its power. Belief systems thrive on being hidden away, buried deep in the unconscious. They grow big and strong on your denial of them, your refusal to acknowledge them.

Locate the belief system in your body. Where does it live? Where do you feel it? In the solar plexus? Lower back? Neck? Jaws? Find it and experience the sensation. What does this belief system feel like? What physical sensations are associated with it? Experience that you carry this belief system in your body.

Label the belief system; put it into words, and feel those words reverberate through the body: "I'm not good enough."

Now, move this belief system out of your body. Imagine those words moving out of the body onto that now familiar distant screen. See them outside yourself. Notice what sensations arise in your body when you do this. As you did with the thoughts, dissolve the words away into golden light. Watch that old belief system become a cloud of golden light—pure energy.

Allow that golden light to return to you as pure energy released from the old belief.

Don't try to force it into new beliefs. Just breathe it in and feel it move through you. Don't try to tell yourself, "OK, that one's gone." Just experience the release and the transformation of an old habit pattern into pure energy. In that moment of transformation, you have freed yourself. You can be sure you'll have to do this exercise many times. You can do it regularly for several days or weeks, or as you feel the need arise, when you are in the grip of the belief system. Don't forget to spend the time breathing in the golden light at the end of the exercise.

Once you've identified several beliefs, you can see how they are all interconnected. You can understand, for example, how "I'm not good enough" leads to "No one loves me," which circles back to "There's something wrong with me." That's connected to "I can't."

Play with the pattern. Write down the belief systems randomly, and draw lines connecting them so that the whole configuration looks like the diagram of a molecular structure. These systems are the building blocks of the conditioned self. As you become free of them, you have much more energy to grow, change, and create.

You can work with the pattern as you did with the words. Imagine the structure you've diagrammed located in the body, and then coming out of the body, onto the screen, and dissolving away into the light. Feel the light return to you as pure energy.

If you are honest with yourself and not concerned only with the obstructive belief systems, you will also discover some positive belief systems. Give them equal time, honoring the resources within you. Repeat them to yourself. Breathe them through you. Acknowledge them with the same wonder as you did the negative ones. Find out where in the body they dwell. Experience the life-affirming energy they carry, and allow it to flow through you and permeate your body.

Releasing Energy Caught in Old Psychological Patterns

I SUGGEST THAT WHEN YOU READ THIS CHAPTER, YOU MAKE YOURSELF A CUP of tea, settle in, and prepare to spend a little time with it. Psychological patterns develop through repeated experience, and shifting them takes time, patience, and constant attention. To have optimal energy for your life now, it's vital to look at how much of your energy may be stuck in past experiences. Releasing that energy is an ongoing process.

Each of us is a collection of experiences. Our childhood experiences teach us how to relate to life; habit patterns we learn in childhood can cause us to feel fatigued or depressed years later. These experiences shape, condition, and define the way we see the world, the way we interact with it, and the way we perceive ourselves. What we think of as the self is a complex set of conditions, experiences, and influences. Our present personality is like a river with many tributaries—many streams that flow into it. There is the cultural stream. We are all a product of history, time, and culture. We cannot separate ourselves from where and when we were born. There is our heredity and our biology, as an individual and as a member of the human race. There is the ancestral/psychological stream—the patterns of behavior, thought, and feeling that are passed down from generation to generation. There are our early childhood experiences, which imprint our energy profoundly. An enormous amount of energy is tied up in old knots of heredity, culture, and family. I often see people who have been in therapy for years, who have explored their patterns from every angle and thoroughly understand the genesis, from a psychological point of view, of certain behaviors, responses, and patterns of relationship in their lives. They have gotten in touch with their feelings, grieved and raged, dialogued with and held the inner child. And somehow the patterns still persist.

There is a point in the inner work where watching yourself is a bit like watching a movie. You see yourself being yourself, doing things you've always done. Some part of you is sitting there, like a member of the audience, saying to the character on the screen, "You know, you don't have to do this. No, no, no, not that guy, not again. Can't you see it's just the same old story; can't you see he's no good for you?" And meanwhile the hero or heroine goes on, playing out her role, caught up in the drama, oblivious to your warnings.

This is a difficult phase. Awareness has deepened and heightened and you can see clearly, but the awareness hasn't yet penetrated the dense energy of habitual reactions.

It is important to emphasize your growing awareness rather than the frustration and sense of failure that arises when you see yourself doing the same old thing. At least you see it; at least you know it's the same old thing. There are patterns you are working with; this insight is an essential foundation for the eventual shifting of behavior. As you become more aware of your awareness, more in touch with the awareness in you that observes the pattern, you develop your power of choice and your ability to consciously move out of the pattern. It takes time! One of the things I have learned in my work with people is respect for the forces we are all dealing with: the power of greed, anger, and ignorance, and the old forces of culture and ancestry. They are strong.

There is a story about the Buddha. When he made the decision to sit down under the Bodhi Tree and not rise until he had become enlightened—until he had seen through and understood those forces of greed, anger, and ignorance—he took a wooden bowl and tossed it in a nearby river. "If I am to become enlightened, let this bowl float upstream." It did. We are turning upstream when we begin developing awareness, shifting old patterns, using our power of choice to reclaim our energy from those old forces, and living from a place of love and compassion and understanding rather than from the old habits of blindness and anger and fear. It takes considerable energy to do this, another reason why we need to learn to work with and conserve our energy. Over and over, we will find ourselves swept away and carried miles downstream by the force of the current, our old way of being, our habits, and our conditioned responses. So over and over, we have to turn upstream again.

Again, please give yourself credit for seemingly small moments of shift, freedom, and choice. If you grew up in an abusive home, feeling the verbal or physical force of anger, living in fear of an explosion, and you yourself have struggled with the legacy and habit of anger, you are working with a powerful force. If you find yourself one day simply looking at your partner, withdrawing the anger, letting it melt away into an energy of love, and letting go for just one moment, that is a moment of enlightenment. It is a taste of the freedom, the liberation that all spiritual traditions emphasize. It's the kingdom of heaven. You may have grown up in a home where no one expressed affection, where everyone was busy with outer activities and no one seemed to have time or energy for communication. You yourself may have learned to deny and repress your feelings. If you now begin to communicate with your partner and express the love you feel to your children—even if it's not perfect, no matter how small it may seem— that's a huge shift. Notice it; give yourself credit; feel the energy that comes from beginning to acknowledge how much you have changed. You lose energy by focusing on how much you haven't changed.

Self-judgment is one of our mostly deeply ingrained patterns. As we work on ourselves, there's lots of opportunity to fall into this old pattern. You might say to yourself, "Why am I still doing this? How can I be so stupid? I understand this backwards and for- wards; what's wrong with me that I can't change? I just want to get rid of this pattern. When is it going to go away?" In my experience, that's one of the biggest illusions and one that costs us a lot of energy. Those old patterns aren't going to go away. They'll shift, becoming less rigid and more fluid. They'll get smaller, less gripping. The awareness, love, and acceptance will get bigger and stronger. The anxiety, anger, and grief will become more like clouds in a clear sky, blips on the screen. But we are who we are. We have had certain experiences, and the power of habit is strong. Certain experiences may always trigger certain responses. A fear reaction that once lasted for years, weeks, or hours, however, may come and go in a few seconds. Eventually, it may not arise at all. If it does—if some old pattern you thought was long gone resurfaces—it doesn't mean there's something wrong with you. It just means you have to re-gather your energy, recognize the strength of the old forces, and make a commitment to yourself to continue doing what you have done a thousand times before: to continue finding new ways of responding to the old pattern.

Human creativity is boundless. Just imagine if all the energy that goes into creating weapons of destruction, time-saving gadgets, and new ways of entertaining ourselves was directed instead toward discovering new ways of being together on this planet, transforming our relationships with each other and the earth. That creativity is there in all of us, waiting to be used for our benefit, growth, and transformation. Releasing the energy caught in old psychological patterns means tapping that creativity and inviting it to work in each of our lives. Your natural human creativity can go to work for you to paint a brighter picture of your life, weave a new tapestry, or tell a different story.

The first step toward this goal is this: Spend a day being aware of your awareness; notice how much you notice. See that you see the pattern, whatever it may be at a given moment, and also see the you who sees the pattern, and so on. This practice is like dropping a pebble in a still pool, producing an ever-widening, deeper circle of awareness that leads eventually to an acceptance of all the parts of yourself. As you see the different patterns—the ways you respond to people and events—and you become aware of your awareness, you begin to realize that you are all these parts, and also that you are more than the sum of the parts. There is a central *you*, an awareness that holds all the parts, sees all the patterns, and embraces the fullness of your self. The more you experience this awareness and identify with it, the less you experience yourself as just this part, or that part, or all the parts in conflict with each other. That awareness begins to take a more central role, gains power, and becomes more active in your life.

From this place of greater awareness, it is possible to work with old patterns. The simplest way to access the psychological patterns, the family imprints, is getting in touch with the child in you. The following exercise can help you encounter that child and release energy that may be caught in old experiences. Please read the entire chapter, though, before you actually begin the exercise. Also, please reflect on this: this exercise is not about reliving the experiences of childhood or digging up old memories. What happens for a lot of people is that as soon as they imagine the child, they identify with it. They'll say, "I feel sad. I feel afraid. I feel lost." Those feelings belong to the child. Your present life energy goes out to the child, in the same way you experienced in the "Reclaiming Your Energy" exercise that your energy can go out to other people. People often over-identify with the child in themselves. For years, they unconsciously play the child in many life situations. Then as they begin to be more aware of the child, perhaps through inner child work, they often get lost in the feelings of the child and become overwhelmed by them. To have sufficient energy for your present life, it is important to reclaim the energy from the child aspect of your being, without abandoning or denying its presence, and to experience yourself as a greater awareness that can embrace the child.

To do this, it is necessary to understand that while the child is a powerful part of you, it is not all of you. There is your adult self. There is the awareness that can hold the child, understand it, love it, dialogue with it, and teach it new ways of being in the world.

Because the child lives in the past, it lives in old feelings. It may be overwhelmed by fear, grief, or self-blame. But again, these feelings are not all the child is. There is a child full of energy, love, curiosity, wonder, and delight. What is helpful is to get that child out of the past, out of those dark places of pain, fear, sadness, and confusion.

Very often in therapy, you have to go back into your past and relive old experiences. This process can be helpful. At a certain point, however, it is also helpful to retrieve yourself from your past. It was through personal work with my therapist, Eleanor Robbins, that I discovered the magic of recovering the child from the past and bringing her into the present.

Recovering the Child

Sit quietly, do several minutes of following the breath and awareness meditation, and then imagine the child you were, whose experience still shapes the way you live your life. See her, or him, at any age—whatever arises. Perhaps it's the child you know from a photograph. See yourself caught in that moment of time. And just be with the child. Notice the thoughts, feelings, bodily sensations, or images that arise in you as you think of or visualize the child.

As you imagine the child, see it as it is in the photograph and draw the line of light around yourself. Separate from the child. Know that you are not the child; any feelings of grief, fear, anger, or confusion that arise in its presence are past. They are old. They belong to the past. Draw the line of light again, feel yourself, and affirm to yourself in any way you can—in whatever words work for you—that you do not have to continue to carry these feelings.

Imagine that the little girl or boy is sitting there in the midst of some scene from the past. Imagine it as a movie; let the scene expand. Maybe the parents are having a fight, and the little boy is alone in his room. Maybe the little girl is at school, and the teacher is mad at her. Maybe she's in a dark room, terrified of the ghosts under the bed. See this scene on the movie screen of your mind. Be aware of yourself as the observer.

Imagine yourself as you are now entering the scene. You, the adult—looking as you do today—appear on the movie screen. What do you do? You may take her hand; you may pick him up. You may talk to him gently; you may tell her a joke. You connect in some way. You may encounter resistance. The child may be afraid or distrustful. It may be happy to see you. Just stay with it.

Eventually, you want to get the child out of the scene. You may carry her out; he may walk with you holding your hand. It's your imagination, so anything is possible; you can teleport, fly, whatever. You bring the child into a place of safety: a landscape, a room, a place of light that you imagine for it.

And from that place, together you watch the old scene dissolve away into a cloud of golden light. You feel the presence of the child, here with you, now. Maybe she's happy. Maybe he's scared. Just hold that presence in your mind, and do your best to maintain your detachment. You're the adult, holding the child. Empathize, understand, love, and soothe. "Shh, it's all right. You're here now. You're here now. I'm with you. I won't abandon you."

Leave the child in a safe place in your imagination, with guardians. Promise to return soon. Draw the line of golden light around yourself, dissolve the whole scene away into golden light, and spend several minutes in awareness meditation, noting your thoughts, emotions, and physical sensations and following your breath. Surround yourself with rainbow light. You may then want to debrief yourself by writing down your experience.

This one exercise is not going to heal all your childhood wounds and release all the energy caught in your old experience. It's meant to assist you in whatever inner work you may be doing. It's one more key to the energy in you that's locked away in the patterns of the past.

As you practice this exercise, you may come up with many variations.

One variation that can be used on an almost daily basis is this: Let's say somebody at work triggers the child in you. He reminds you of your father and plays that role over and over. You go into a room with him, and you're five years old again, tongue-tied, afraid, inwardly angry, and overwhelmed by feelings of helplessness. Before you go to work, in your imagination, visit the child in yourself in that safe place you have created for it. See the landscape or the room in rich detail. Imagine windows, trees, toys, colors, or light. Embrace the child. Reassure it: "I'm going to work, not you. You get to stay here in this great place and have a good time. I'm the adult, and I'm the one who's going out there and dealing with that guy. You don't have to. And he's not your father. He's just this guy I have to work with."

Usually, the child in you wants to know that someone's in charge. This is especially true if as a child you did have to take charge! As you detach from the child, taking care of it but not identifying with it, you increasingly have the sense that someone *is* in charge—that you have a choice. You don't have to dissolve into tears or go into silent rage in the face of "that guy." You can draw the line, be aware of yourself, return any negative energy that's coming your way, and deal with the situation.

People also carry landscapes, environments, rooms, and houses in their memories. The environments of childhood make a deep impression on us and hold a lot of energy. Think for a moment of the settings of your childhood. Is there a particular house, room, or place that appears? If it has a negative energy, you can meditate with the image, seeing it on a distant screen, and allowing it to dissolve away into golden light. If necessary, make sure to retrieve the child, as in the exercise above, before dissolving the scene away.

You may encounter a resistance to dissolving away these old scenes or to bringing the child forward. People often say they want to let go of the past, but they are not so eager when they are presented with the opportunity to tangibly, energetically do so. Once again, the sense of self is identified with the old experiences, painful though they may be. Exercises that work with the child in you can be framed by meditations of self-inquiry. After you have attended to your child self, you can place that aspect of yourself in context by sitting with that spacious question, Who am I? Who is it that has all these experiences? What is it that holds and loves this child in me? The answer comes, not in words, but in a gentle breath of tenderness, a whisper of light, a melting of the heart. You are the child, and you are that loving awareness.

People often discount the effects of their childhood experiences on their energy because they didn't have traumatic childhoods. They compare themselves to people who have been terribly abused and think they don't have any right to be so angry, fearful, or sad, because their childhood wasn't really so bad. What matters is honoring the experiences of the child. How often is a sensitive child told, "Don't be afraid; there's nothing to be afraid of"? People keep telling themselves this, and maybe inside they keep being terrified. The child in you may simply need to hear that it's okay to be afraid: "You're afraid. I may not understand what's making you afraid, but you are. It's okay." Children don't understand the complicated language of therapy. The child in you needs to be communicated with in simple, straightforward, reassuring terms.

Sometimes, people feel helpless because they simply can't remember much of their childhood. Whether you remember your childhood or not, the child is there every day, reacting to situations in your life. You can feel the child in you—afraid, angry, confused, excited, or shy—in many situations. You can connect with your childhood by experiencing how the child in you reacts in the present. A greater awareness grows, releasing more energy: "This is the child in me reacting to this situation. I am not only the child. I have choice. I have options. The child didn't, but I do."

We've glimpsed the tip of the iceberg in this chapter. The child in you has a huge reservoir of energy, energy that may have been stuck in fear or anger, shoulds and shouldn'ts. There are many ways to work with this child and your old psychological patterns. Perhaps you are beginning to see how the exercises work together. Reclaiming your energy from people in your past, for example, can help to release the energy caught in old psychological patterns.

When you work with yourself in this way, you are working with energy, and energy is real, tangible, and actual, not just "imagination." Modern physics teaches us that a seemingly solid object—a chair, for example—is in fact, from another perspective, a collection of energetic patterns. So are you. This is why these meditations hold so much potential for change. They help you to reshape and redefine your experiences, and the structures and patterns of your consciousness.

Depending on your own past experiences, these meditations may best be done working with a therapist you trust or a guide of some kind such as a friend or partner. This one chapter certainly is not intended to take the place of ongoing therapy; rather, it is designed to support it. If you are just beginning to get the idea that a lot of your energy could be tied up in old psychological patterns, or if you struggle with childhood trauma, please seek the help a qualified counselor can offer. If you are in therapy, you can consult your therapist before doing these exercises.

Keep in mind that we often hold a lot of energy in two seemingly contradictory beliefs. One says there's no help out there; you have to do it alone. The other says you can't do it alone and you have to have help; somebody else knows what's best for you. Neither belief is the complete truth. The universe offers a great deal of help—from people, spirit, our own higher selves, and nature. Sometimes, we need that support and need to ask for it. At the same time, there is an aloneness everyone experiences, a place or a time where no one can do it for you. It's up to you.

Part of the beauty of these meditations is that you can do them alone or with others as you see fit.

Transforming Anger into Positive Creative Energy

....

IN THE HINDU TRADITION, THE DARK GODDESS OF CREATION AND DESTRUCTION is called Kali. She is the great cosmic mother, terrible and beautiful, beyond good and evil, full of primal energy. She creates and destroys. She destroys that which obstructs us, our illusions, our blindness. She brings vision and understanding. By destroying our old selves, she births us into new life. Traditionally, she is shown with one of her four hands dispensing blessings while another dispenses destruction.

In Tibetan Buddhism, there are many powerful spirit protectors known as wrathful deities. Legend has it that when Padmasambhava brought Buddhism to Tibet, he subdued the local evil spirits and transformed them into protectors of the dharma (Buddhist teaching). In Japan, the Buddhist temples often have carved guardian figures of fearsome aspect.

Jesus Christ preached love and nonviolence, yet when he was confronted with the moneylenders in the court of the temple, he overturned their tables and denounced them.

Anger is a powerful energy in each of us, a fact of human existence that cannot be denied, repressed, or willed away. It can be transformed from a hurtful, destructive force into a positive creative energy. This fact is recognized in the stories and teachings of almost all spiritual traditions.

Contemplations on Anger

In working with anger, we will use the meditative method of contemplation. It is possible to reflect on, explore, and study your anger; you can know it intimately, understand it, and dialogue with it. To approach one's anger contemplatively is already a radical shift in energy. Inviting your anger into a calm, contemplative space that you provide for it in your consciousness begins to give you a different perspective, a different experience of anger.

Blind, uncontrolled anger is a destructive and hurtful energy. Many people have learned to be afraid of it. It's important to be with your anger when you're not angry to get to know it. Meditate with your anger. Most people don't think of meditating with anger. It's not your usual meditation practice. Try it. Take time to contemplate your anger.

Contemplation is a form of meditation; it is very different from thinking about things over and over. You have to create a contemplative space. Then as you begin to explore your anger, the energy is similar to reading a book, very slowly, turning the pages, really absorbing every word, trying to understand. In contemplation, you are reading yourself—turning the pages of your experience, absorbing your own knowing, seeing your reflection, and studying yourself.

Begin by contemplating in this way. Consider these possibilities: I do not have to get rid of my anger. I do not have to repress or deny my anger. I do not have to be controlled by my anger. I do not have to hurt others with my anger. I have the choice to transform my anger. Anger is powerful life force energy. I can use this energy to support my life.

Tomorrow, or the next day, or whenever you feel moved to do so, light a candle, sit down, and surround yourself with the clear light of awareness. Invite your anger into that clear light. Tell it you want to know it better; you are not afraid of it. Notice what images, thoughts, feelings, and sensations arise. Explore them. What kinds of things make you angry? Are there patterns there—recurrent situations that trigger anger?

How do you express anger? Do you tend to explode, or do you turn it on yourself? Are there specific people in your life now or in the past who you are angry with? What are your feelings about anger? Write all this down if you wish. Dialogue with your anger. What does it want to tell you?

Don't try to do anything with all this information. Don't expect miracles. Just explore.

As you meditate with your anger, return occasionally to your breath, to the thought, *This anger can be transformed. It is pure life energy.* When you are done, thank your awareness for being present, and thank your anger for being willing to dialogue with your awareness.

On another day, contemplate the nature of anger in a general way as you meditate. People are ashamed of their anger, or they feel justified in it. It's a very personal thing. Take a meditation period to step back from it and examine it from a universal, philosophical point of view. Question it. Probe it. What is anger? Where does it come from? Is it bad? Good? Can you experience its universal nature, see how it arises according to causes and conditions? Can you experience it as pure energy?

When you choose, contemplate your anger as a mirror. The basis for this contemplation is, Whatever makes me angry in another person or in the world is a reflection of something in myself. How do I see this quality in myself?

On another occasion, you can again work with a particular recurrent situation that arouses your anger. Sit down, follow your breath, and enter into meditation. Imagine the situation; explore it. Reflect on the concept that anger is power. How do you need to use your power in this situation? What choices do you have? What does your anger want you to do? Often, anger is impelling us toward action. Imagine acting out different choices. How do you feel in each situation?

For example, there may be someone you know who makes you angry. You could use some of the earlier exercises to detach your energy—to stop reacting to and losing energy to this person. Or perhaps you need to confront him or her. Is there a mirror for you? Something you need to see about yourself? Is it actually abusive? Do you need to act to protect yourself? There are many choices in any given situation.

The contemplations described above can be very useful for those who are trying to get in touch with their anger. Pounding pillows and screaming doesn't work for everyone, and people often find that while catharsis feels good, it doesn't automatically transform the anger; it doesn't always affect one's habitual reactions. Reflecting on and exploring the nature of anger and one's own personal experience with it can help anger to emerge.

In your contemplation, think of the stories told at the beginning of the chapter, from three of the world's great spiritual traditions. These stories tell us a great deal about the positive aspects of anger. In Kali, we experience the acceptance of anger as part of who we are. We are both light and dark. We have our shadow sides; we constantly experience creation and destruction in our lives. We are born and we die. It is impossible to deny the destructive force of the universe. The earth has its tidal waves, earthquakes, hurricanes, and floods. So do we. Our inner storms sweep through us, breaking up old fears, old ways of being. Anger, when it is acknowledged, worked with, and experienced as pure energy, can be cleansing.

Just as Kali teaches us acceptance and understanding of anger, so the Tibetan deities represent another powerful aspect of anger. Often when we are angry, we are trying to protect ourselves. If we are attacked, we want to fight back. The instinct to defend ourselves, loved ones, or our territory is ancient and deep. Anger can be a way of defining oneself, setting a boundary, establishing one's energetic territory. Teenagers often use it in this way. This protective, territorial aspect of anger is another theme for contemplation. If there is a recurrent situation that makes you angry, ask yourself, "What am I trying to protect or defend? Am I really being attacked, or does it just feel that way?"

The exercise of creating a boundary can be helpful when one feels attacked. You may need to work with detaching and protecting your energy with psychic protection and shielding. You may find that the child in yourself is feeling threatened. Perhaps a current situation triggers some old fears and anger. Does the child in you need protecting? Use the exercise in "Releasing Energy Caught in Old Psychological Patterns" to work with anger that is triggered from childhood experiences.

In your contemplation, you can imagine your anger as a protective figure—a knight, a mother tiger, a shining light, whatever works for you. Honor that protective energy, thank it, and ask it to continue to protect you. The metaphor of the wrathful deity carries an intense energy of transformation. The negative, draining, destructive energy of anger can be transformed through awareness into a powerful protection.

In the story of Jesus, we experience another face and voice of anger: righteous anger, which has the power to motivate and provides the energy to confront injustice and oppression. This is the anger that arises not from the desire to control and dominate, nor from a feeling of powerlessness and frustration. This is the anger that demands change; it is the anger that awakens. This anger we need in this world.

Reflect on this kind of anger. How do you experience it in yourself? Can you experience your anger as a motivating force? Again, what is your anger telling you to do? Feel the power of anger that has in it clarity, wisdom, and a clear voice that says, "This is not all right. This needs attention. This needs action."

Also contemplate power and powerlessness in relation to anger. Explosive anger allows people to feel momentarily powerful; repressed anger creates a sense of powerlessness. One day, as you meditate with anger, allow yourself to feel the physical sensations of anger in your body. Think, *I am angry*. Breathe that thought through your body. Remember the experience of anger; notice what happens in your body. Notice the power of anger to choke, to grip, to create tension, numbness, heat, and waves of energy in the body. Whatever you experience, acknowledge the power of anger and ask yourself: "How do I choose to use this power in my life?"

Sit with the sensations in the body until they subside; imagine them as pure energy, available to you to support your life now.

This whole chapter, or sections of it, can be read as a contemplation of anger. If you wish, you can set aside a day, a week, or a half hour a day for a week with the intention of meditating on your anger. Create a contemplative space, breathe quietly, read a portion of the chapter, and reflect on the issues and questions raised here. You can write down your insights and experiences meditatively, reflectively. Feel and absorb what you are writing and breathe it in. You will find that the awareness of anger that comes to you under these circumstances will begin to arise under other circumstances. Your experience of anger will change. Your habitual reactions will begin to change: you'll associate anger with the meditative state of mind. You will release the energy of the anger to work with you and for you. It will help you to act and communicate clearly.

If you've spent time contemplating your anger when you aren't angry, it is more likely that your awareness will be present when you are angry. Awareness will arise in the midst of the habitual reaction. Your inner voice will say, "Wait a minute. What's really going on? What do I really need to do here? What are my choices?"

It takes discipline to meditate with your anger in this way. People often want their meditation to be a relief, a release, a period of calm and silence. Anger is perceived as a negative, disturbing energy. It's a simple fact that most people would rather spend hours going around and around in their anger, being angry and talking about how angry they are, and at whom they're angry, than spend fifteen minutes when they're not angry actively working to transform their anger. The choice is yours.

Fear as Energy

....

YOU PROBABLY KNOW WHAT FEAR FEELS LIKE. IF YOU DON'T, PLEASE FEEL FREE to skip this chapter. Chances are that you are familiar with the pounding heart, the sweaty palms, and the dry mouth of fear. Perhaps you know how it tends to dwell in the solar plexus; you have experienced that feeling of the pit of the stomach just falling away, sinking into nothingness. You may be even more familiar with generalized anxiety—the sense of unease, discomfort, and nervousness that seems to have no particular cause.

Fear arises from a variety of sources. There's fear that's just a response to sensed danger in the outside world. Watch a deer, a cat, or a dog suddenly become aware of a perceived threat. The entire body tenses; all the senses go on alert. It's the fight-or-flight response. There's fear that's a learned response. Some children spend their childhoods tiptoeing around the adults in their life, never knowing when the anger will explode, when the blow will fall. Fear becomes habitual. One learns to wake up with fear, to fall asleep with fear. This chapter is not about discovering the root and source of fear, but rather about experiencing it in a different way—transforming it into pure energy. Again, please read the whole chapter before doing the following exercise.

Transforming Fear

Sit down meditatively, center yourself, and summon the feeling of fear. As with anger, it's best to do this at first when you're not actively experiencing fear. Invite the feeling of fear into your consciousness. Remember what it feels like. Pay particular attention to the physical sensations. Where does it dwell in your body? Where does the fear get stuck? It may be in the solar plexus; there may be a tightening in the chest; there may be tingling in the palms of the hands. Just stay with it, allow it to be.

Tell yourself, "This is simply energy."

Breathe into it. If you find yourself overwhelmed by the sensations, get up, walk around, get a drink of water, and put the experience aside until you can practice the exercise again with a friend or healer present.

If you stay with the sensations, they will shift, melt, move, and begin to flow. You will feel waves of energy pass through your body. You may feel warmth or tingling. Simply experience the energy. As the energy flows, a feeling of peacefulness arises. The breath comes more slowly and evenly. Saliva begins to flow. Say to yourself over and over, "This is just energy, energy moving, energy that is available to me to live my life, to do what I want to do."

You may experience alternating currents of peace and fear. The energy may settle and then suddenly return to its old state, with all the physical sensations. Stay with it as long as you choose. Then get up, drink some water, and move around. Surround yourself with golden light. You may feel peaceful. You may feel uncomfortable. When energy begins to move, it is not always comfortable. The movement may lead you deeper into the other emotions that are often associated with fear: anger and grief. Take time to experience what arises.

Affirm: "Fear is energy. I can use that energy in a new way."

Think of something you want to do or create in your life and direct the energy toward that vision.

If you experience panic attacks, it is best to do this exercise with an experienced therapist or healer. It can be very helpful to remember that panic attacks hold a huge amount of energy. To learn to experience a panic attack as pure energy, and to hold your awareness in the midst of it, can transform your experience of it. Usually, a panic attack is intensified by the fact that people are afraid of the attack itself because the energy is so intense. There is a fear of being overwhelmed by it. The fear of the attack then intensifies the attack.

Fear is energy. In its pure form, it is your life force energy gathering itself to respond to a threat. Its purpose is to protect you. If you experience a lot of fear or generalized anxiety, you probably need to work regularly with the exercises of setting a boundary and psychic protection.

Earlier, I mentioned the flight-or-fight response. Fear, like anger, is impelling you to action. And yet people will say they are paralyzed by their fear. If you experience a lot of generalized anxiety, nervousness, streams of small fears in relation to daily life, or bigger fears about accomplishment, success, or expressing yourself, movement will help. Dance every day. Go for a walk, run, exercise, play tennis. The message of fear is, *Move!* Don't stand still and don't get stuck. If you're thinking about something you want to do, someone you have to talk to, or something you're afraid of doing, and you feel stuck, get yourself up, shake out your body, and go for a walk. The energy that is released by the movement will then help you to do what you're afraid to do—maybe today, maybe tomorrow, maybe a week from now.

Walking meditation is a great way to combine the meditative approach described in the first exercise and fear's demand for movement. Instead of sitting down, go outside and find a path where you can walk slowly and meditatively. Anchor your vision on the ground, on your feet taking steps. Feel your feet on the ground. Pay attention to your breath, and begin to walk slowly. Feel every step. Take a breath with every step. Notice the support of the earth, and thank it. Breathe in. Breathe out. The earth will anchor you; it will ground you. Walk for as long as you like. You can also alternate walking and running.

Or you may want to find a tree, sit under it and ask it to absorb your fear. The earth, the trees, and the sky will carry away your fear, if only for a moment.

You can experience a shift in how you experience fear. You can feel the energy behind it. You can stop identifying it as something that paralyzes you and keeps you from doing what you want. You can experience it as an energy that wants you to move, that wants to protect you. Don't expect miracles. Fear isn't going to disappear from your life. You can change your relationship to it. It can become a helper. The little miracle is that for one moment—today, now—you can experience that transformation.

Releasing Energy Through Self-Expression

THIS PRACTICE IS SIMPLE.

Whatever you have always wanted to do to express yourself, do it, and do it often. Sing, dance, write, play, draw, talk to people, embrace people, go for a walk and sit under a tree, climb a mountain, tell a story, knit a sweater, paint a picture, laugh, cry, write a poem—or a novel or an article—take a trip, buy a new dress, paint your living room, make love in a different way at a different time, go on a meditation retreat, study astrology—or computers or high finance—build a house, make a sculpture, work with wood, learn a language, create a ritual…

From the dawn of human history, people have sung, danced, told stories, and sat together in circles around fires below the vast night sky. They have cried and laughed. The life force longs for expression. To be fully here, in this human body, is to allow that life force to flow—to move, to speak, to sing. Do it alone, with other people, or in a class, anywhere, anyhow. Your energy will thrive and grow. The more you express your creative energy, the more you will have.

Don't wait. Today, begin to do a little of what you have always wanted to do. Don't think you don't have time. Sing on your way to work. Dance while you make dinner; write for five minutes before you go to bed. There are no excuses. Life has room for life, even in today's stressful world. If some physical limitation keeps you from doing something you used to love to do, find something else.

And once you've begun to do a little of something you've always wanted to do—try doing something you never thought you'd do!

Love as Energy

LOVE IS ENERGY. LOVE SUPPORTS, AFFIRMS, AND MAINTAINS OUR ESSENTIAL life energy. Love is something we always want more of. We can receive love from others, we can give it to ourselves, and we can experience its universal presence.

Love is a presence in the universe. It is here, now, with you, breathing with you, moving with you, thinking with you. It can be invited into your life. Ask it: "Please, love, come to me, be with me, and let me experience you."

People are often told to love themselves, and they haven't got a clue how to begin. Here's a tangible way to do it. You can spend a few minutes when you wake up in the morning or before you fall asleep at night loving yourself.

Loving Yourself

Lie still and breathe in love. Remember a time you felt really loved and loving; bring the experience of love into your consciousness. Then put your attention at the top of your head. Love your head: your hair, your brain, the bones of your skull, your eyes and ears, your nose and tongue. Move your attention through the head, giving it love, feeling love for all these specific aspects of your unique self. Notice where you feel obstructed. Maybe you've never liked your nose. Do your best to simply hold it in your consciousness with love.

Move through the body in this way. Pay attention to every organ, to the veins and arteries, to the nerves and cells. You may find your attention span for loving yourself is brief. You'll get to the throat and find yourself worrying about what you have to do tomorrow. Bring yourself back to yourself. Notice what you experience: the resistances, the fears, the encounters with parts of yourself you've never liked. You'll see that love flows easily sometimes, and sometimes it takes work. You enter into relationship with yourself, commit to loving yourself, by doing this simple exercise.

When love flows easily, we have so much energy. When it seems blocked, we feel drained. The more you can let love move in you—invite it into you—the more it will flow, the more energy you can have. Here's another way to do this. Use your imagination.

The Presence of Love

Imagine that all you are is a vessel, a container for the presence of love. Love expresses itself through you and experiences itself in you. When you touch things—as you pick up a book, put down a cup of tea, wash a dish, or touch the hand of another person— imagine that love is passing through you. Love is touching, reaching, holding. Feel the tenderness in your hand for the things you touch. When you move, love moves. When you speak, love speaks.

This is not an exalted spiritual state, attained only by saints and gurus. It is an experience open to all of us. When you experience it for a moment, be grateful. Don't try to hold onto it. It won't last, but it will return.

Love brings us energy, but these days it feels as though there are so many blocks to just loving. Let's explore some of those blocks together; let's contemplate them, and then at the end of our contemplation there will be more meditations for experiencing love.

One of the questions that I hear most often is this: "How can I love if I cannot trust? I have been hurt so many times. I am afraid of being abandoned."

Please be aware, first of all, that the one person who can never abandon you is you. Make a deep commitment to yourself: No matter what, I will stay present with myself.

I will love myself. I will take care of myself. Your breath is a wonderful symbol of this commitment, this love for yourself. As long as you are you, in this physical form, your breath is always with you, supporting and nourishing you. When you feel unloved, unloving, and therefore in a low energy state, stop and experience your breath. Feel how it nourishes you. Feel your own breath as love full of life-giving energy. As you experience your breath in this way, you renew your commitment to yourself; you stay present with yourself; you do not abandon yourself.

Do you have to wait until you can trust completely to love again? Life's experiences teach us to be wary of people, to know that people can be aggressive and hurtful. People want to open their hearts and love unconditionally, but their inner awareness says, "Be careful. Be aware. Keep your eyes open." We have learned only by painful experience not to trust everyone. Don't deny that learning. Only experience with a person will tell you whether you can trust her. Even if someone is completely reliable and there for you, circumstances may take him away. You can't know the future, and you can't wait for absolute assurance that someone will always be there and never hurt you before you love. By its very nature, love involves risk, uncertainty, and the possibility of loss. If you want more love in your life, you have to open yourself to confusion, sorrow, and pain as well as to joy and pleasure.

Love is confusing. I hear many people say, "If I could just get clear about my feelings for this person, it would be so much easier." Accept it. Human love is not clear. To open one's heart means to accept ambiguity, confusion, and mixed feelings. An open heart is willing and able to be joyous, full of love, angry at times, confused, and even hurt. It is able to demand, and to give up its demands. It asks, gives, receives, reaches out, and retreats. There is a tenderness that comes from knowing that you can't always be clear; there is a relief and a release of energy.

Sometimes, we learn early in our lives to love someone who is not good for us. If, during childhood, we wanted the love and approval of a parent who was not able to give it, we can spend our whole lives seeking love where we are not likely to find it. Or we can become aware of the difference between love and the attraction to that which is old and familiar. In working with the exercises in this chapter on loving yourself, you become more familiar with the feeling, quality, and energy of love. As that familiarity grows, you begin to look for that experience in your relationships with people. You begin to be attracted to that energy in others.

People seek to give and receive unconditional love. Ask yourself, Is this realistic? A lot of energy is lost in holding others and ourselves to an impossible ideal. Perhaps unconditional love comes from the Divine, from God, and from Mother Earth. Perhaps our human love is almost always conditioned by our conditioning, whatever it may be. We do get glimmers of that divine love in ourselves, in moments of complete acceptance and embrace. They are beautiful, energizing, and nourishing, but human beings have needs and desires. Ongoing relationship with another has to acknowledge this fact. Unconditional love does not mean pushing aside our needs and desires because we are uncomfortable with them or afraid to express them.

In today's world, however, a potential block to loving another is the growing belief system that your intimate partner is supposed to meet all your needs. People come to me with a catalogue of all their needs that are not being met in relationship. It's certainly important to explore what needs are not being met and how to address these needs with one's partner. It's also important to reflect on this: perhaps love is not about meeting needs. Perhaps that is the inner child speaking. We're in trouble if we expect the other person to be Mommy or Daddy and give us everything the actual Mommy and Daddy didn't. Love sometimes means giving up the idea that the child in you will ever get everything it didn't. No matter how much love you get, that child's experience will continue to arise and influence your response to your partner. Ongoing attention to the child in yourself (see "Releasing Energy Caught in Old Psychological Patterns") helps you to distinguish between the child's needs and the desires and needs of the adult in adult relationship.

Also in today's world, people are searching for meaning, fulfillment, purpose, empowerment, and support. Quite often, they look for all of that in intimate relationship. This places a huge strain on intimate relationship. While relationship is a profound-spiritual path—a way to grow, open, let go of ego, and experience oneness—it is only one way to do so. To be intimate with another, we need to be intimate with ourselves and also feel our connection with something greater than ourselves. We can experience our partner as a manifestation of the Divine, but if we expect him or her to be God, then we're in trouble.

One of the biggest fears many people have about loving another is the fear of losing themselves in the relationship. So many people have had the experience of giving themselves up for another, losing their identity for the sake of keeping the love of another, whether it's a parent in the past or a partner in the present. Many of the people I encounter are what I call mergers. These are highly empathic people who are sensitive to the feelings, thoughts, and needs of others. Usually, they have learned early in life that this empathic merging—knowing and responding to the needs of others before those needs are spoken—is what love is. Often mergers will get lost in the dominating and needy energy of a parent, or if the parent is emotionally unavailable, the child feels a desperate hunger for connection and union.

Mergers need to learn that merging with another is not the same thing as love. To enter into union with another, to truly experience that another is no other than your own divine self, is a beautiful experience. It's important not to confuse this experience of oneness with the daily challenge, pain, and joy of living with and loving another person. Knowing and defining yourself, and being able to acknowledge and accept the unique self of the other, are essential tasks of loving. The exercises in setting a boundary, reclaiming your energy from others, and returning energy to others can be helpful for empathic people who tend to lose themselves (and therefore their personal energy) in relationship.

At the same time, many people are so afraid of giving up their identity that this fear blocks their capacity for relationship. In any ongoing relationship, sometimes you have to surrender to your partner and vice versa. You can do this consciously, from a deep knowing of yourself and the other, without giving up your identity. It's a delicate balance, and there is no formula for knowing when to stand your ground and when to surrender. That's why continued self-exploration and self-knowledge form the foundation for a healthy intimate relationship.

Buddhism teaches that there are two aspects to this world and this human life.

These are called the absolute and the relative, the great formless oneness and the world of form. The absolute is our oneness, our interconnectedness. We are all one universal energy: you, me, the chair on which you sit, the air you breathe, the tree outside your window. We all share this universal energy. Mystics have experienced this energy since time immemorial. From this absolute point of view, our love for another grows out of the recognition that we are one, that there is no separation between us.

From a relative point of view, I am I and you are you. The chair is the chair. The tree is the tree. That universal oneness never manifests itself exactly the same way over again. Every manifestation of the oneness is its own unique pattern, unrepeatable, precious, and complete in itself.

To love deeply is to experience oneness and at the same time recognize and appreciate the uniqueness of the other. It is the ongoing challenge of discovering and affirming your own uniqueness and that of the other. To love means to truly see the other, to cease imposing your vision, your ideas, and your way of being on the other. Love is dialogue, exchange, and communication between one unique Other and Another.

Here are exercises that can help you experience both the absolute and relative aspects of love.

Merging and Emergence

Breathe quietly, close your eyes, and imagine the presence of someone you love—an intimate partner, a divine being, a friend, a child, an animal. Surround that being with golden light. As you breathe, imagine that you and the other melt away, dissolving into a great sea of white light. Or the other melts away into a cloud of light, and that light merges with you and you melt away too. Or you melt into the other. Feel that wonderful letting go, the merging into and floating in the sea of light. You are surrounded by the energy of love, supported by it.

Then, with your breath, come back to yourself. Take a breath, feel your body, draw the line of golden light around your unique self. Bring the other back into form. See his or her unique form reemerge. The golden light becomes a flame in your heart and in the other's heart. Surround yourself and the other with rainbow light. Spend some time with that individual form, observing it, noting its unique qualities, and appreciating it. Note the color of the eyes, the way the hair grows, the individual characteristics you know so well, whether physical, emotional, or mental. Include the ones that drive you crazy.

Thank this other being for the gift of its presence in your life.

Two people can do this together. It's a way to learn to move back and forth between the experience of union with another and the experience of separateness and individuation. Alternate between experiencing each other as pure light, formless unity, universal energy, and as two unique beings, appreciating each other's differences.

You can also do this meditation with an image of the Divine: Mary, Jesus, Kuan Yin, Buddha, Tara, or Shiva. You can do it with a tree, an animal, or a flower. You can do it with your reflection in a mirror or a photo of yourself. You can do it with the whole earth.

Imagine the earth as one sees it in the photographs taken from space: a beautiful blue-green-white sphere floating in a vast darkness. Imagine that you, this earth, and all the planets and galaxies are merging into one great white light, as a universal energy. Feel that universal energy throbbing in you, breathing through you. Imagine yourself, the earth, the galaxies, and the planets all returning to their separate forms. Feel the love, the tenderness, the energy that arise as you return, as you see everything in this universe as your very self, and everything in this universe as the Beloved, the divine Other.

Often people feel alone, and the feelings of loneliness, isolation, and alienation drain energy. You are never alone. The whole universe breathes love, support, and affirmation. The meditation above can help you experience how much love you have even if you are not in an intimate relationship. People ask over and over, "Why am I alone? Why can't I find a relationship that works?" There are so many reasons why you might be alone. Perhaps you need to learn that you are truly never alone. Perhaps you have chosen solitude for this reason. Or are you afraid of losing yourself in relationship? You may be lonely at times, but do you truly want to be in relationship with all its demands and potential pain? Love is a mystery. It comes to each person in a unique way, in a breath, a whisper, a moment. Your best friend's experience of love will not be the same as yours. As you explore your way of loving, you come to know yourself better.

The more we experience the love we have, the more we open ourselves to receiving and experiencing a greater abundance and flow of love in our life. Enter into meditation. As you breathe in, feel the presence of love entering you, nourishing you, penetrating to every cell in your body. As you breathe out, breathe out love. Imagine love going out into the world, carried by your breath to every corner of the universe. Breathe in the presence of love. Use your imagination. Imagine that with every breath love is pouring into you, soaking into you.

Prayer as Energy

....

FOR MILLENNIA, PEOPLE HAVE PRAYED. THEY HAVE PRAYED INDIVIDUALLY; they have prayed together. They have prayed for things, for enlightenment, for health, for safety, for the well-being of loved ones, for blessings. They have prayed for visions, to know, to understand the will of God, to submit to the will of God. They have prayed for the victory of their side, the defeat of the other. They have prayed selflessly and selfishly.

When you pray, your prayer joins with every prayer that has ever been said. As soon as you say a prayer, you join a vast community; you participate in an experience that goes back to the beginnings of human history.

A lot of energy can come from prayer, but what is it? How do you define it? This chapter is a contemplation of the nature of prayer, intended to help you find your own form of prayer, to open the energy of prayer for you.

Think about what prayer means to you. You may have a prejudice against prayer: it may mean to you people praying for things or a lot of hypocritical people asking God for blessings on their enterprises. Such prayers may seem to come only from ignorance, greed, and anger. Whatever prayer means to you, take a moment to let go of that concept. Even if you pray all the time and think you have a pretty good idea of what prayer is, take a moment to simply explore and define prayer.

What is Prayer?

Prayer is dialogue with the Divine—with that great consciousness that bears so many names in this human world and ultimately cannot be named at all. Prayer is dialogue, communication, listening, asking, and naming. Prayer is stillness, being with what is.

Prayer is a bridge between the formless and the form, the absolute and the relative. Almost always throughout human history, prayer has been addressed to a form, an intermediary, Mary, Jesus, gods and goddesses, saints, spirits.

To pray is to express your willingness to listen to a greater consciousness. To pray is to acknowledge that you are not alone, that there is something greater than yourself that listens, receives, and gives.

Prayer is affirmation. It affirms the presence of God, or whatever you choose to call the Divine.

Prayer is a particular state of consciousness. It reflects your relationship to the Divine. Traditionally, one kneels to pray, with the hands folded. Reflect for a moment on that posture. Adopt it. Stop reading and take that traditional posture of prayer. Feel the energy in the posture. In the hands joining, there is the bringing together of all dualities into a unity, and the offering of those dualities to the great unity. In kneeling, you come close to the ground and connect with the earth. The hands together, folded or pointing upward, form the connection between heaven and earth. In prayer, you are drawing down energy from heaven to earth; the energy travels, earth to heaven, heaven to earth. You are the conduit, the means by which the universal consciousness manifests on earth. The posture of prayer is essentially the posture of connection, connecting form and formlessness, divine and human.

The posture of prayer signifies one's willingness to be a conduit, a vessel. The posture of prayer is a focusing, a directing of the divine energy. That focusing can be done for a particular purpose; healing, for example. One is directing the divine energy through one's own conscious intention for the benefit of another. So prayer is calling, intention, and focus.

Experiment with the posture of prayer, and see if different postures enhance your experience. As the body adopts different positions, the consciousness transforms in response. Another traditional posture of prayer is to open the hands and arms, lifting them wide, palms up. Try that now. Still from the kneeling posture, just raise your arms up and out, with the palms of the hands open, and feel how you receive from the universe. The energy streams in, and you hold it like a chalice. You offer it where it is needed.

Another posture of prayer is prostration, in which you kneel further down, lower your head to the ground, and extend your arms on the ground. In this posture, you feel yourself prostrate before that which is greater than yourself. This is not a posture of humiliation; it is one of recognition. It is a posture of great power. In prostration, you blend with that which is; you do not stand up or out, or alone. You are a part of the whole. Your individuality merges with the whole. Try it.

It can be very transforming just to experience these postures, but don't do them automatically. Feel what's going on. In the posture of prayer and prostration, there is great energy, peace, serenity, and surrender. And, actually, it isn't necessary to adopt any particular physical posture. Prayer is an attitude, a posture of consciousness in relation to the Divine.

Prayer is healing. People ask, "How can a prayer possibly heal?" More and more scientific studies are demonstrating the healing power of prayer,[10] and still no one can say exactly how or why it works. No one can define or quantify the healing power of prayer. If we begin with the belief that we all share our existence in a universal energy, then it makes sense. In this universal energy, perhaps time and space do not exist in the way we think they do. In that great web, everything is connected to everything else. So just as a mother reaches out with love to touch her child when the child is sick, so the energy of our prayer perhaps follows the lines of our energetic connections and touches the illness, injury, or hurt in another person with love and healing. Prayer focuses your energy, giving it intention. In Tibet, prayer flags flutter everywhere in the wind. The belief is that the wind carries the prayer written on the flag far and wide. Think of that when you pray for someone. Your prayer carries the energy of love to that person.

Prayer is a form of remembering. One of the primary characteristics of the human mind is that it forgets. It forgets what it is, what it is a part of. It forgets love. It forgets what it has learned and understood. Prayer helps us remember that we have a connection with the Divine, a connection to energy greater than our own personal energy.

Prayer is talking to God. It's as simple as that. Sometimes, people will adopt a particular form of God to talk to. Prayer is conversation with God. Talk with God regularly. God has many names, so use the one most personal to you, the one with which you feel the greatest connection. This conversation begins to shift the belief system that you are alone—that if God exists at all, it is a reality that is somehow far away. Many people feel separated from the Divine. As you converse with God, you bring that presence into your life. It becomes tangible. Prayer is the tangible experience of God, and it brings you energy.

If you believe, as many do, that everything around you is a manifestation of God— that God is no other than that universal energy—then everything you do is prayer. Your life is a constant conversation with God. When you speak with other people, you are conversing with God. When you touch something, you are touching God. When you walk down the street, you are walking with God and are surrounded by God. Many people find it possible to have glimpses of this state of prayer; few people live in constant conversation with God. But ask yourself this question sometimes when your energy is low: "At this moment, can I see the Divine in myself?" And sometimes, when you feel another person draining your energy, ask yourself, "In this moment, can I see God in this person?" It isn't easy, but it's possible.

Prayer can be asking for things. There's nothing wrong with asking for things; however, the old saying "Be careful what you wish for, because you may get it" is a good one. So if you are going to pray for a particular outcome, it's good to do it with awareness; ask for the greatest good for yourself or for another. If you feel something is missing in your life, don't be afraid to ask, to pray for it, to say, "Dear Divine Mother, dear God, dear Universal Spirit, dear Whoever, I ask for your help in manifesting this in my life. I ask for the support of the universe in bringing this into being. I ask for the blessing of the universe." If you ask in this way, it acknowledges that you play a part in the fulfillment of the prayer.

You can also ask in this way: "I offer this prayer to the universal energy flow. May it enter the stream and manifest for the greatest good."

In prayer, you come together with the Divine. You and God work together in partnership. The outcome is the result of that partnership in action. Whenever you pray for something, look: What are you doing to bring that into being? Feel your hand in the hand of the divine presence, the Great Spirit, God, Goddess, the universal consciousness in whatever form works for you. Dialogue with it. Ask. Put forward your question or your need. And then listen. In the moment, answers or insights may come. Silence may surround you. A blessing may come, and a tangible, palpable sense of lightness may descend on you. Then keep listening. As you move in your life, notice: How is this prayer being answered? Again, it doesn't always come as you expect, but there's always a response. Learn to recognize it. Bring your awareness to that question: How is my prayer being answered?

Communication is always happening in this universe. Listen to the birds, how they sing to one another. Every single aspect of the animal kingdom communicates. The plants stir in the wind. The molecules of oxygen that enter the body through the breath join with other molecules. Neurotransmitters are always transmitting. We live in a world of constant communication. The universe is always communicating. Prayer develops your skills in understanding what it is saying. In the birdsong, there is a message. In the blue sky or the cloudy sky, there is a whisper. In the sound of the wind, the feel of the rain, there is information. In your breath, there is knowledge and wisdom. All these messages bring energy to us if we pay attention to them, if we let ourselves receive the energy. Sometimes, an answer to a prayer is simply a tree branch moving in the wind or a raven flying overhead. To pray is to be in communication with all that is.

I once met an old woman, in India, one early morning by the side of a dusty road leading out of a timeless village at the foot of the sacred mountain Arunachala. She was carrying a pitcher of milk and a bowl of fruit and flowers. I watched as she stopped by a stone figure of the god Rama. She offered the flowers and fruit to him. And then— carefully, lovingly—she bent down and poured a dish of milk for the small stone cat next to him. I came back the next day, and there she was again, feeding the cat of the god. She had a relationship with Rama and his cat. These were no stone figures to her; they were God. This is prayer.

Rumi, the twelfth-century Persian mystic, refers to God as "The Friend." [11] The more we converse with this Friend—the more we experience the presence of this Divine Companion and enter into intimate relationship with The Friend—the more energy we have.

Acceptance as Energy

....

SOMETIMES, NO MATTER WHAT WE DO, HOW HARD WE TRY, HOW MANY decisions we make, what teachings we follow, or how much we work on ourselves, circumstances remain difficult, our energy stays low, our minds and bodies or other people overwhelm us. We've all had this experience. These are the times we gain energy by surrender, the acceptance of what is. We lose energy through guilt, self-blame, resistance, and wanting things to be different.

The basic awareness meditation (see "Awareness as Energy") is a good, simple way to open the door into the acceptance of what is. As you sit quietly following the breath, turning the attention to the arising and ceasing of sensations in the body and thoughts in the mind, you are in the present moment, being with what is.

Acceptance means letting go of all ideas you have about how things should be. You can experience this letting go in a tangible way in a meditative state. As you practice the awareness meditation, turn your attention to the tension in your body; notice the areas of tension and practice releasing that tension. Breathe gently into it and feel the letting go, or feel how you hold on. Simple relaxation tapes can be helpful with this practice.

Or, as you practice the awareness meditation, place your hands palm up on your knees. Clench your hands into fists, then open them and feel the letting go. Practice feeling the difference between holding on and letting go. As you breathe quietly and experience the contrast, you can affirm to yourself, "I accept what is," or "I let go," or "I am not in charge. I can't control what happens." Use whatever words work for you.

Very often, using methods such as those offered in this book becomes another way of trying to control things, and there are always situations in life where we have to admit that we are not in control. The universe is a vast web of interacting forces and energies, and to think that we can understand it completely and therefore control what happens to us can be very frustrating. People are often told that they create their own reality; therefore, if things aren't going well in their lives, they think something must be wrong with them, and they end up judging themselves severely. There are external circumstances. We are always in interaction with the greater universe. We may have choices about how we respond to external circumstances, but we can't control them. There's a difference.

In my work with people, one of the most common questions that arises is simply "Why?" People want to know the reasons for their pain, frustrations, illnesses, and difficulties. This is understandable, and it can be helpful to look at karma, psychology, cultural influences, or spiritual lessons. Ultimately, we often come to a place of silence, acceptance, and surrender to the great mystery; we recognize that there is a bigger picture, and perhaps the question "Why?" can never be truly answered.

The following meditation can help you come to that place of surrender and acceptance, letting go into the universal energy flow; it will help you remember that you are a part of that flow, not an isolated individual in control of what happens. It's a meditation for the times when you've come to a wall, when you don't know what to do, when nothing is working. It's also a meditation for every day, for opening yourself to the guidance that is always there.

Star in the Heart

Sit down quietly. Breathe. Feel your frustration, your pain, your confusion, your deep knowing that there is nothing you can do. Slowly bring your attention to your heart center. Perhaps it hurts, is tense, or feels constricted. Be with whatever is there; don't judge it.

Imagine a small seed of white light, a point of light in your heart. This seed expands into a star. The point of light radiates beams of light in every direction. It looks like the star the wise men saw over the manger when Christ was born. Visualize it, feel it, or tell yourself it's there, whatever works for you. Be with it. Spend time with it. Let it shine in your heart,

This star represents what we are all seeking: the great Truth, the Source, the Whole, the Divine. It represents your inner knowing. For centuries, people steered by the stars and knew their connection to the heavens. There is a powerful metaphor in this meditation. You surrender your personal will, recognize yourself as no other than this great cosmos, and feel the universal energy within yourself. This star represents an inner compass. The light in the darkness is always there; it guides you and supports you.

Meditating with the star can bring the peace of surrender. "Not my will but Thine" is the spirit of this meditation. Usually people think of this greater will as God's will. You can experience it that way, or you can experience it as surrender to the great mystery of this life and the universe. You can experience it as simple acceptance of what is, a letting go of resistance and battle with the circumstances of life. The greater will is that light in your heart. As you connect with the light in yourself and give it space to shine in your life, so much energy can come to you.

The Dance of Energy

....

LIGHT STREAMS THROUGH THE WINDOW. IN THAT RAY OF LIGHT, THE DUST in the air, ordinarily invisible, dances. There is a dance going on around us constantly—a dance of energy. The leaves on the trees dance in the wind. Our thoughts dance in our mind.

Imagine for a moment that nothing in this world is solid. It is all a big field of dancing golden particles of light, like the dust in the sunlight. You are surrounded by energy in motion even as you think you walk on solid ground.

Close your eyes and imagine this dance of energy. The more you think this way, the lighter you become and the more energy you feel. You begin to discover you can dance with things, events, and relationships. The dance is a perfect metaphor for human relationship and for life.

In different situations, ask yourself, "How can I dance with this?" This difficult person, your car breaking down, waking up tired in the morning. Hold out your arms to your partner of the moment, whatever or whoever it may be. Follow the rhythm of the moment, the music of the day.

Remember that all forms of intentional movement can increase your energy level dramatically. Walking, dance, yoga, tai chi, tennis, rowing—it's your choice; each is an opportunity to increase your energy. Life is motion; it never stands still. As you experienced in the "You Are Energy" meditation, even when you are sitting in meditation, your body is in constant motion.

It's a great practice to sit in meditation, feeling the energy pulse within you, being with it until that very energy lifts you up. You may find yourself dancing, or spontaneously moving into a yoga posture you have been doing for years, or dropping the ball into the basket with unexpected precision, but now it's coming from deep inside. Also try the reverse: dance your heart out, and then sit down and feel the silence reverberate around you. Notice how you settle into meditation more easily; feel the tingle and rush of energy throughout your body. Movement and meditation go together; they enhance and support each other.

Sometimes, people ask, "What can I do with my anger? My fear? My grief?" Dance it. Truly, literally, dance it. It's what people have always done. Put on some music and move, by yourself, in your room, in your garden. Dance your anger, your fear, your love, your longing. As you dance, you become one with the primal dance of energy— the eternal dance.

Connecting with the Universal Source

....

YOU RECEIVE ENERGY FROM THE FOOD YOU EAT, THE AIR YOU BREATHE, YOUR sleep at night, and the exercise you do. Yet you know, from your own experience, that you also receive energy from a variety of intangible sources. Certain experiences can give you energy: watching a sunset, viewing a work of art, enjoying a concert, having a conversation with a friend, or being with someone you love. The exercises in this chapter are designed to help you discover your personal connection with the vast sea of energy surrounding you, so that you can replenish your personal energy from this universal source.

Begin by reading and contemplating this statement, quoted from the book *The Holographic Universe*, by Michael Talbot: "When physicists calculate the minimum amount of energy a wave can possess, they find that every cubic centimeter of empty space contains more energy than all the matter in the known universe." [12]

How amazing! The universe is full of empty space, and that empty space is full of energy. We exist in a vast and infinite sea of energy. If we begin with this premise, that empty space is full of energy, the question "How can we access that energy?" becomes "How can we enter that empty space?" Through our minds, in our consciousness, we have the opportunity to experience that empty space full of energy. By going within, we can access the universal energy.

The Space Between

To enter into the empty space within your mind, begin by following the breath. Don't try to control it; simply notice the inhalations and exhalations. Become aware of the space between your breaths—that infinitesimal fraction of a moment between the in-breath and the out-breath. Allow that moment to expand. Don't try to hold your breath; relax into that space. Allow your thoughts to dissolve into that space, and to continue to dissolve as you slowly exhale. Breathe slowly but normally, shifting your attention from the breath itself to the space between the breaths.

When you have done this for a while, shift your attention to your thoughts. Notice the stream of thoughts, and then try to notice the space between the thoughts. Thoughts come and go, but there is a space, a whisper of silence, between the arising of one thought and another. Explore that space; focus on it, return to it. Notice how spacious your awareness becomes as it dwells for one moment in that silence between one thought and another.

We learn to pay attention to things, people, places, thoughts, and feelings, but we can also learn to pay attention to that vast empty space that surrounds, holds, and provides the background for all things to exist. Next time you look up at the night sky, instead of noticing the stars, notice the empty, dark space. Enter into it. The more you pay attention to space, the more you will have of it, and the more energy you can experience.

In general, begin to pay attention to the spaces between, your transitions. When you drive from one place to another, you can use that time to energize and refresh yourself. Play a tape of quiet music, and as you listen, be aware of your breath, the sky, the sounds of traffic—and, of course, your driving! Set the intention "I am going to use this space between one thing and another to restore my energy." While you are standing in line at the bank, become aware of that moment as a space between. When you are finished with a meeting, a phone call, or a particular task, take a few moments to close your eyes and enter into empty space before you go on to the next thing. As you do this practice, you are constantly accessing the energy of that empty space throughout your day and replenishing your energy from the vast universal storehouse.

When you want to enter the empty space quickly during the day, visualization can make it more tangible and easily open the gateway to that spacious consciousness. Close your eyes and briefly visualize the night sky full of stars, or a bright blue sky with white clouds drifting by. Experience that great sky as your awareness, that which experiences all the passing events, thoughts, and people of your life. Affirm "I am the space between the stars, the great blue sky." Breathe in the space. The more you enter into the greatness, vastness, and spaciousness of your own mind, the more energy you will have.

There are other images and meditations that can help you connect with the universal sea of energy. When we are in the womb, we experience a direct connection with an energy source greater than ourselves. Through the navel, blood, oxygen, nourishment, and life energy are continuously flowing into us from the mother. At birth, we are separated from this source; we instantly have to find our own source of life—our own breath. But even now, as adults, we can experience relaxation, an increased flow of energy, and a feeling of nourishing ourselves by imagining energy coming directly to us through the solar plexus, a main nerve center in the body.

Golden Light Meditation

Lie down and place your hand on your navel, the palm gently cupped over the area. Imagine warmth and light in that area, and breathe quietly. Imagine the universal energy as a golden light all around you, a cloud of golden light that fills the room and surrounds you. You are connected to that cloud of light by a cord or tube of light that comes directly from your belly button. Feel the warmth and light travel from the navel upward into the chest, down into the belly, and through the legs. Lie there as long as you like, allowing that golden light to nourish you. As you open your eyes and breathe deeply for a moment, know that this energy source doesn't really go away. You may experience it whenever you choose.

This is a wonderful meditation to do before you fall asleep at night. Then, of course, you don't open your eyes. You simply drift off to sleep surrounded by the universal energy, fed by it and connected to it. If you follow this exercise by surrounding yourself with rainbow light, then you protect and conserve the energy you have replenished.

In doing this exercise, you can think of a mother and her child. In this meditation, you are the child of the Divine Mother, nourished by the energy from which all things grow. If you have a good relationship with your mother, this meditation can help you reconnect with that experience. If you felt unloved by or disconnected from your biological mother, this exercise can be healing and energizing because it gives you a chance to experience the universal mother energy. You can have the energetic experience of being nourished that you were denied as a child.

Another contemporary and practical metaphor for this meditation with the golden light is that of the car and the gas pump. You take your car regularly to the gas station to fill it up. In this meditation with the golden light, the universal energy pumps into you as gas pumps into your car, only the universal energy doesn't cost you anything, and you aren't draining the earth's resources. All you have to do is remember that this energy is available to you, and open yourself to it.

This Beautiful World as Energy

....

FOR THIS PRACTICE, YOU DON'T HAVE TO USE YOUR IMAGINATION. GO OUTSIDE and take a train, a bus, a car. Walk. Find trees, grass, sky, rock, water. Trees on a city street are fine. A park, a mountaintop, an ocean or a desert, a cloud outside your window—it doesn't matter. The natural world radiates an energy that you feel as soon as you bring your attention to it.

In the Hindu tradition there are spiritual gatherings called *darshan.* The word means simply to be in the presence of a holy being. The belief is that simply by being with a saint or a great teacher, one who has experienced the presence of God, we experience the grace of God, the energy that flows from the Divine. The natural world is imbued with the divine energy. Darshan is available to you daily, right outside your door.

Darshan

The very next chance you have, take the darshan of a tree. Find a tree, in a somewhat quiet place, and sit beneath it. Ask for its blessing. Feel its energy, its silence. Imagine that the tree is pouring light down on you and through you. It may be a translucent, spring-like, green light, or autumn gold, or winter white. In every season, trees radiate energy, healing, and balance.

Take the darshan of clouds and sky, flowers, rocks, streams, the ocean, a hill, the mountains. As you experience every single aspect of nature as sacred, you are receiving darshan everywhere.

Notice the birds, the clouds, the wind. Experience the shifts in your energy that come with changes in the weather. You don't have to live in a remote place or go into the wilderness to stay in touch with the seasons, the elements, the animals, and the plants. It's easier out of town, but it is possible in the city.

Through photographs, you can receive the darshan of the Himalayas, the Andes, the jungle, the ocean, the desert—all the remote power places of the world. Some of the energy of a place is transmitted through the visual image. Try it. Some night when you're too tired to do anything else that's in this book, take down a book of photographs of beautiful, remote, wild places. Turn the pages slowly. Don't get distracted by planning trips or feeling bad that you don't have the time or money to get to these places. Just soak in the energy. Perhaps the book is a photo album with pictures of places you've been. Through your memory, invoke the energy you felt in those places; relive the experience.

The earth and sky surround, uphold, embrace, and nourish us. Sometimes, people have conflicts about being here on this earth, in this body, with other people, struggling with all the endless details and issues of human existence. Most of the world's religions encourage us to look beyond this world for salvation. The following meditation can help you experience this world as a source of energy. It is similar to one of the meditations found in the chapter on love, but not identical.

Gaia

Follow the breath for a few moments. Imagine that you are seeing the earth from a great distance. See it as from space. How beautiful it is! Green, blue, white, shifting light and shadow, ever-changing colors. On this fragile, translucent sphere, so many stories are being played out. Feel the self that lives on this earth—the self that plays out your individual story—and become aware of that awareness that sees the whole, from the perspective of space. You are the great awareness that embraces the earth and stars and space, and you are also you—body and spirit, blood and feeling.

Recognize this distant earth, floating in space, as your teacher. This sphere of floating green, blue, and white light is a great teacher, an unparalleled master. Honor this teacher; bow to her. Know that you are blessed to live with her, care for her, and learn from her.

Imagine now that you come closer and closer to the earth. Land. Feel your feet on the ground, here, now. Look at your hands and love them. Stretch your body. Feel yourself at home on earth.

Breaking the Downward Cycle

THERE IS A CYCLE THAT OCCURS WHEN YOU DON'T FEEL GOOD—WHEN YOU ARE tired and drained by people and events in your life, by chronic physical conditions, or by depression. If you experience chronic low energy, fatigue, depression, anxiety, or pain, you know this downward cycle well. Everyday events become increasingly stressful, and other people don't understand this. You went to the grocery store today, big deal. It is a big deal! It takes a lot of your precious store of energy to get out the door, deal with people, drive in traffic, and make small decisions. Feelings of powerlessness, over-whelm, and fear set in, intensifying the fatigue and low energy. You don't have the energy to do the things that might help. You try one therapy, medicine, or supplement after another, and you lose hope. This book promises no miracle cure, but it can help, little by little, day by day, as a valuable adjunct to other approaches. If you're in that downward cycle, here's how to use this book.

1. Don't even try to actually do the exercises. Just read them, a little at a time. After you read a chapter, lie down, close your eyes, and just drift. Allow thoughts, feelings, or images from your reading of the chapter to float through your mind. Let the possibility that you can have more energy arise in your mind. Breathe in these thoughts: *It is possible. Things can change. I can feel more energy.* You are probably tired of trying to do things to make yourself better, so just let

yourself receive energy from what you read, rather than immediately feeling you have to do something more.

2. These are the most important exercises for you:
    *   The Rainbow Wash
    *   The Rainbow Shield
    *   You Are Energy
    *   Setting a Boundary
    *   Releasing Energy Through Choice
    *   Connecting with the Universal Source: The Golden Light Meditation
    *   Acceptance as Energy: The Star in the Heart.

Do these exercises as often as possible. They don't have to be done at a special time or in a special way. You don't have to do them exactly. Just remember to surround yourself with rainbow light as often as possible. You'll find that color can nourish your energy just as food nourishes your body.

3. If you haven't already done so, get some outside help. It can be, for example, a therapist, a pastor, a massage therapist, a support group, a nutritionist, an acupuncturist, a doctor, a bodyworker, or a spiritual healer. It has to be someone you see regularly, a minimum of once a week if possible. When you leave the person, you should feel nourished and sustained and have a little more energy, even if only temporarily. Be sure to explore with a health practitioner you trust all possible physical causes for low energy, and address those issues. It's hard to break the downward cycle alone; needing help is not a weakness.

4. That support at times may be medication. Many people take antidepressants, hormones, and other medications to address low energy, fatigue, and depression. Often, those who are trying to heal themselves, who are drawn to alternative health approaches, will either deny themselves this help or feel guilty about taking

medication. While medications can be abused and overused, they can also be useful tools to shift one's energetic balance. These days, our systems deal with numerous stresses and toxins. It's not easy to maintain a biochemical balance. If you find that a particular medication helps you to stabilize your body-mind system, don't be afraid of it. Be sure to have a doctor's guidance, and be aware of possible side effects. Don't self-medicate, and especially don't go on and off a medication without a doctor's guidance. If you and your doctor decide on a particular medication, take it with a little ritual, acknowledging its help and asking it to help you have more energy for your life. Don't rely on it alone; continue to pay attention to diet, exercise, and working with your mind.

5. Let go of self-judgment and self-blame. Few experiences drain your energy more quickly than these two states of mind. Letting go of these states is easier said than done. Use the meditations in this book to help you release them. The chapter on "Thought as Energy" can be particularly helpful with this.

6. Highlight small changes. It is a big deal when you feel good for a day—when you have enough energy to accomplish what others might see as a small task. If on the next day you seem to lose your energy again, recognize this may be the pattern for a time as your energy increases. That's the time for the star in the heart and for remembering that if you felt good yesterday, you can have that experience again soon. Feel good about feeling good, but don't try to hold onto it.

7. Promise yourself that as you start to feel better, you will remember to take care of yourself and use your renewed energy wisely. Often, people build up their energy just a little and then expend it all.

8. Read the affirmation at the end of the book often. It's for you.

Affirmation

....

THIS AFFIRMATION IS FROM ME TO YOU, FROM THE DEPTHS OF MY HEART and my experience.

I believe this entire universe is a sea of energy. I believe in the universal energy that connects us all in the great web of life. Within me, within you, within each seed and flower, each moment, each day and night, that universal energy is always present.

I know from my own experience that the gateway to that universal energy is found in my own mind. As I turn my attention within, I experience whole new realms of awareness and energy. This experience is open to us all. It is open to you, right now, at this moment.

Read the following words aloud to yourself, imagining this is a message to you from that universal energy. Then put down the book, sit or lie comfortably, close your eyes, and let the words reverberate in you. May these words, and all the words of this book, nourish your body, mind, and spirit—today and always.

Yes. Yes. Yes.
You are surrounded by light, embraced by light, nourished by light.
At every moment you are connected to the great Source of your being.
The universal energy flows into you,

Bringing you harmony, energy, and balance
In body, mind, and spirit.
The universal energy sustains and supports you,
Affirms your unique being, your precious life.
Yes. Yes. Yes.

Afterword

....

THE EXERCISES IN THIS BOOK ARE SYNTHESIZED FROM MANY SPIRITUAL AND psychotherapeutic traditions: traditional Buddhist meditations, active imagination, metaphysical studies, traditional methods of psychic protection, my own psychotherapy, and my spiritual healing work with others. I spent the years from 1970 to 1985 in intensive Zen practice and study at the Rochester Zen Center with Roshi Philip Kapleau, author of *The Three Pillars of Zen*. After I left the center, I continued to receive teachings in the vipassana and Tibetan schools of Buddhism. I also acquired a Masters Degree in Social Work and received additional training in family systems therapy. In 1995 through 1996, I received private instruction from experienced teachers in traditional methods of psychic protection and working with spirit. Since 1994, my spiritual path has led me to encounters with the Divine Mother in many forms; in this process, I have experienced the energy that comes from grace and prayer. I continue to practice awareness meditation. The Buddha's teachings are my foundation.

Since 1986, I have conducted individual and group Awareness sessions in the United States and Europe. An Awareness session is an intuitive reading that helps people see, understand, and shift the old patterns of behavior they carry and come to greater self-knowledge. The exercises in this book have been developed during twenty years of work with people; they are the exercises that have proved to be most effective in my practice.

More meditations and information can be found at *www.youareyourpath.com*.

Notes

1. Lynne McTaggart, *The Field: The Quest for the Secret Force of the Universe* (New York: Quill, 2002), p. xiii.

2. See Fritjof Capra, *The Web of Life: A New Scientific Understanding of Living Systems* (New York: Anchor Books, 1996).

3. Joseph Campbell, *Historical Atlas of World Mythology: Vol.1: The Way of the Animal Powers* (London: Times Books, 1984), p. 269.

4. See Francesca Freemantle and Chogyam Trungpa, *The Tibetan Book of the Dead* (Boston: Shambhala, 1971).

5. Pema Chodron, *Start Where You Are* (Boston and London: Shambhala, 1994), p. 36ff.

6. See McTaggart.

7. John Main, *Word into Silence* (New York: Continuum, 2001), p. 53.

8. See Thomas Ashley-Farrand, *The Healing Power of Mantra: Using Sound Affirmations for Personal Power, Creativity, and Healing* (New York: Ballantine Wellspring, 1999).

9. Main, p. 50ff.

10. See Larry Dossey, *Healing Words* (San Francisco: Harper San Francisco, 1997).

11. Coleman Barks, ed., *Rumi: The Book of Love* (San Francisco: Harper San Francisco, 2003), p. 102.

12. Michael Talbot, *The Holographic Universe* (New York: HarperPerennial, 1991), p. 51.

Bibliography

Ashley-Farrand, Thomas, *The Healing Power of Mantra: Using Sound Affirmations for Personal Power, Creativity, and Healing*, New York: Ballantine Wellspring, 1999.

Barks, Coleman, ed., *Rumi: The Book of Love*, San Francisco: Harper San Francisco, 2003.

Campbell, Joseph, *Historical Atlas of World Mythology: Vol.1: The Way of the Animal Powers*, London: Times Books, 1984.

Capra, Fritjof, *The Web of Life: A New Scientific Understanding of Living Systems*, New York: Anchor Books, 1996.

Chodron, Pema, *Start Where You Are*, Boston and London: Shambhala, 1994.

Dossey, Larry, *Healing Words*, San Francisco: Harper San Francisco, 1997.

Freemantle, Francesca, and Chogyam Trungpa, *The Tibetan Book of the Dead*, Boston: Shambhala, 1971.

McTaggart, Lynne, *The Field: The Quest for the Secret Force of the Universe*, New York: Quill, 2002.

Main, John, *Word into Silence*, New York: Continuum, 2001.

Talbot, Michael, *The Holographic Universe*, New York: HarperPerennial, 1991.

Acknowledgements

....

I WOULD LIKE TO THANK THE FOLLOWING TEACHERS: ROSHI PHILIP KAPLEAU, founder of the Rochester Zen Center; Eleanor Robbins, LISW, psychotherapist in private practice in Santa Fe, New Mexico; Marya Low, psychotherapist, trance medium, and shamanic practitioner, Albuquerque, New Mexico; Dr. Robert Weisz of the Milton Erickson Institute of Santa Fe; Mother Meera; the many teachers in the Tibetan Buddhist tradition who give freely of their wisdom to all they encounter; Tu and Láné Moonwalker, spiritual teachers of Universal Beingness; and Holly Curtis, Nia Blackbelt instructor.

Gratitude also goes to my mother, Leslie McCammon; my father, Allan Thomson; and to the two greatest teachers of all: my husband, Bob Schrei, artist and healer; and my son, Joshua Schrei, writer, performance artist, musician, and yoga teacher.

The following people have supported my work over the years both in the United States and in Europe, giving generously of their time, energy, and space: Judy Adnepos, Sabine Bends, Hélène Boitel, Ellen Goldstein Bernitt, Harvey and Linda Feldstein, Malou Fischbach-Zenner, Dale Goldstein, Jan Goldstein, Ellie Hartgerink, Lee Johnson, Nancy London, Rafe and Rose Martin, Michele Matossian, Nancy Miller, Gary Milczarek, Lorin Parrish, Cliff and Patricia Passen, Margrit Schwendimann, Ruth Schmidhauser, and Sibylle Sülser. To all of those I have seen in Awareness sessions over the years, I offer my gratitude for our shared journeys of exploration in consciousness, and for the process that allowed these meditations to emerge. Special thanks go to my friend Alece Carrigan, who connected me with Sentient Publications, and to Connie Shaw at Sentient Publications.

Index of Meditations

ABOUT THE AUTHOR

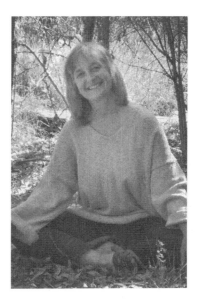

Donna Leslie Thomson is a meditation teacher and a therapist. For fifteen years, she was a student at the Zen Meditation Center in Rochester, New York, under the direct guidance of Roshi Philip Kapleau, author of *The Three Pillars of Zen*.

Thomson has a Masters in Social Work and twenty years of experience in therapeutic work. She teaches the workshops *Awareness Meditation, Meditation with the Divine Feminine, The Vibrant Life,* and *Meditations for Therapists and their Clients*. She has taught meditation and counseled people in Germany, Switzerland, Luxembourg, and the U.S. With her husband, Bob Schrei, Thomson is the originator of SourcePoint Therapy, an energetic healing system.

She has written several other books, as well as a chapter for *The Complete Guide to Buddhist America* (edited by Don Morreale and published by Shambhala in 1998). *The Vibrant Life* has been translated into German.

Donna Thomson resides in Santa Fe, New Mexico. For more information, please see her website, *www.youareyourpath.com*.

Sentient Publications, LLC publishes books on cultural creativity, experimental education, transformative spirituality, holistic health, new science, and ecology, approached from an integral viewpoint. Our authors are intensely interested in exploring the nature of life from fresh perspectives, addressing life's great questions, and fostering the full expression of the human potential. Sentient Publications' books arise from the spirit of inquiry and the richness of the inherent dialogue between writer and reader.

We are very interested in hearing from our readers. To direct suggestions or comments to us, or to be added to our mailing list, please contact:

SENTIENT PUBLICATIONS, LLC

1113 Spruce Street
Boulder, CO 80302
303.443.2188
contact@sentientpublications.com
www.sentientpublications.com

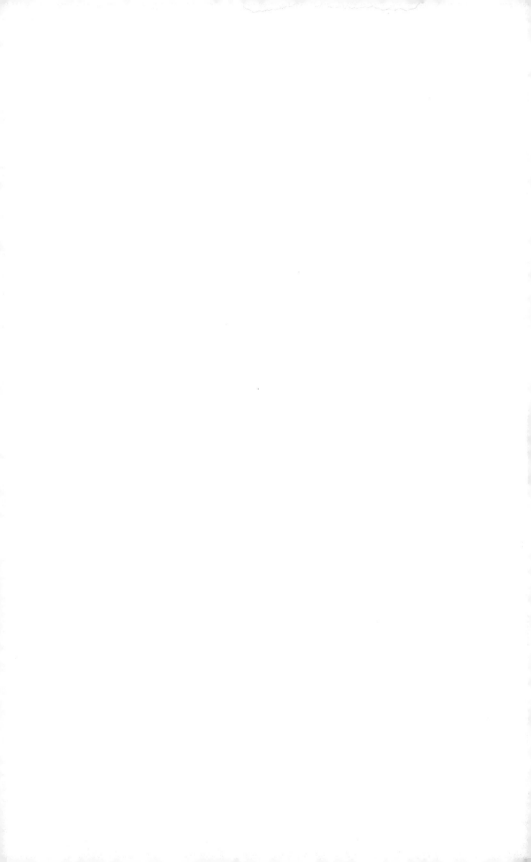